Yoga for Women

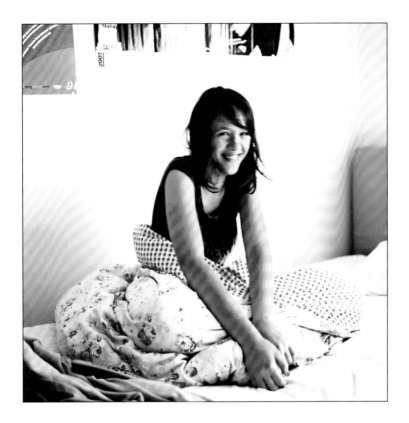

This book is dedicated to my daughter Mira Stina
– my biggest yogic challenge and love.

Yoga for Women

Gain Strength and Flexibility, Ease PMS Symptoms, Relieve Stress, Stay Fit Through Pregnancy, Age Gracefully

BY KARIN BJÖRKEGREN

Skyhorse Publishing

Skyhorse Publishing books may be purchased in bulk at special discounts for sales promotion, corporate gifts, fund-raising, or educational purposes. Special editions can also be created to specifications. For details, contact the Special Sales Department, Skyhorse Publishing, 307 West 36th Street, 11th Floor, New York, NY 10018 or info@skyhorsepublishing.com.

Skyhorse® and Skyhorse Publishing® are registered trademarks of Skyhorse Publishing, Inc.®, a Delaware corporation.

Visit our website at www.skyhorsepublishing.com.

10 9 8 7 6 5 4 3 2

Library of Congress Cataloging-in-Publication Data is available on file.

Cover design by Theodor Jikander, AB Normal
Cover photo credit: Anneli Hildonen

Print ISBN: 978-1-63450-559-8
Ebook ISBN: 978-1-5107-0166-3

Printed in China

Introduction: Yoga and I

I took my first yoga class when I was fourteen years old. My sister Stina took me to Bert Yoga Johnsson at his basement space by Hornstull—yes, that was his name back then, nowadays he calls himself Bert Yogson. We used to go there twice a week for a few semesters. I am not sure if that was when my search for happiness and health was awakened, or if I always had it in me.

I'VE BEEN TO GROUP THERAPY, COUPLES THERAPY, conversational therapy, family counseling, and I've tried the Rosen method bodywork treatment. In fact, I've probably tried every kind of alternative medicine treatment, from colon hydrotherapy to energetic healing by the laying on of hands. I've visited fortune-tellers, mediums, and healers both in Sweden and abroad. I have always had a desire to get to know myself better and to become my own best friend, but most of all to be content with who I am. I want to age with grace and stay healthy and strong for as long as possible.

I was thirty-six years old when I discovered Ashtanga vinyasa yoga and I immediately fell in love. Prior to that, I had tried Kundalini yoga, laughter yoga, different types of meditation practices, and Hatha yoga, just to name a few. At the time I was an extremely stressed out single mom and editor in chief at a magazine with a tiny budget. Stressing and working overtime was normal to me.

My first Ashtanga vinyasa yoga teacher was a forty-four-year-old woman, Britta. Oh my, was she good-looking and fit! I decided then that I wanted to become like her. My intention was superficial, but it soon changed as I embarked on the journey. No matter why you begin practicing, the self-reflection will show up like a letter in the mail. Yoga is not merely a way to exercise your body. Through daily practice you will cultivate a connection between body, mind, and heart. Yoga shortens the distance between the brain and the heart, the mind and the soul. This distance is sometimes called the world's longest yard.

We have been focusing on exercising our bodies to achieve a beautiful exterior for a very long time, but the hunt for the perfect body can sometimes widen the gap between body and mind. Perhaps that is why yoga has become so popular in the West over the last few decades.

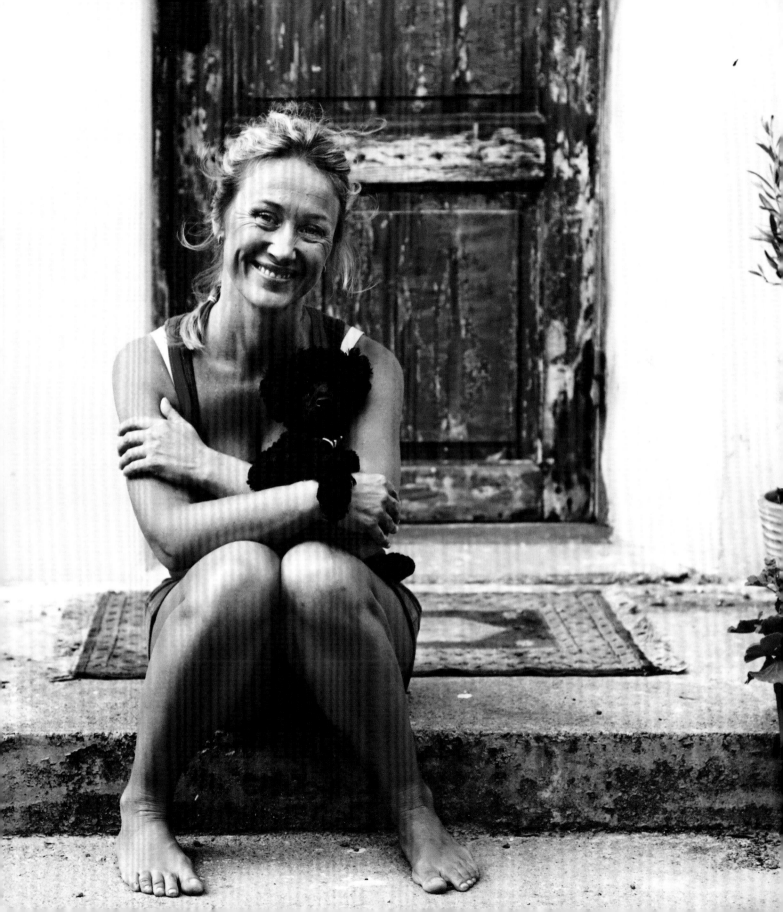

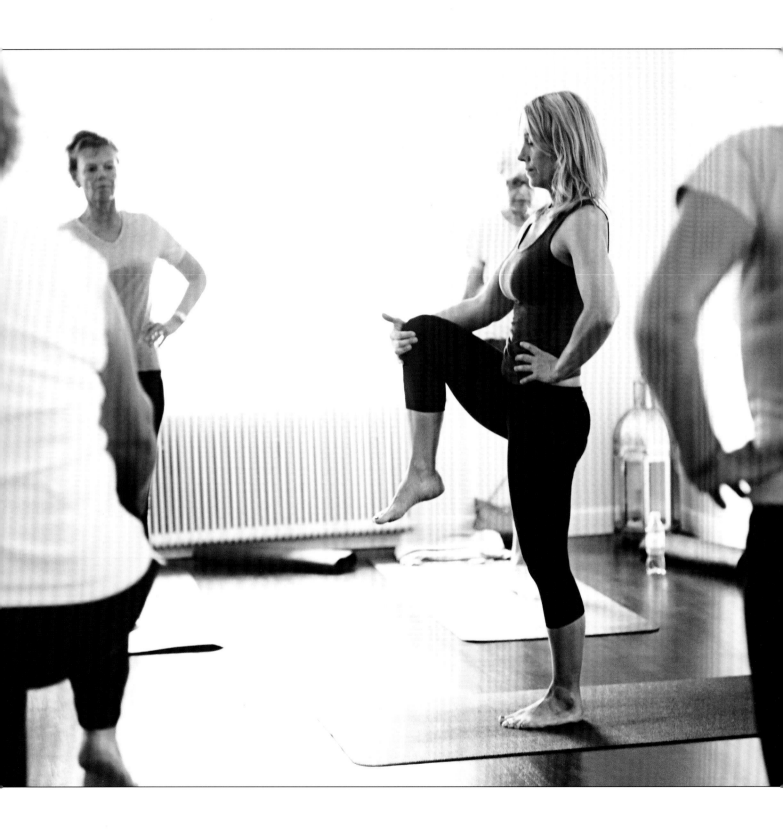

THANK YOU!

The women that demonstrate the yoga poses in this book are all yoga teachers of the ages that the chapters are geared towards. Unfortunately all the wonderful female yoga teachers that I've encountered through the years couldn't participate. However, I'd like to thank you all for sharing your knowledge and for inspiring other women to practice yoga.

So thank you Lotta Bertilsson, Viveka Blom Nygren, Maria Boox, Charlotte Lindström, Gittan Hendele, Therese Fridh, Annelie Bohman, Naomi Grosin, Marie Öfvergård, Lisa Laler, Thomasine Hindmarsch, Margareta Burenstam-Linder, Lina Keller, Dena Kingsberg, Dona Holleman, Johanna Ljunggren, Hilda Norberg, Sofia Noren, Sassa Lee, Marika Bergström, Gwendolyn Hunt, Tina Pizzimento, Britta Lee-jones, Zoiyla Ravanti, Marla Menakshi, Anne Nuotio, Anna Rinnman, Sarasvati, Cecilia Wikner, Gabriella Pascoli, Anna-Karin Sixten, Elizabeth Welsh, Jenny Lindgren, Camilla Håkansson, Carina Fernström, Anna Björk, Marie Stangel, and thank you all you other beautiful yoga teachers that I have not met yet, but who continue to spread the joy of yoga like glitter over your students.

I also want to thank all the male yoga teachers that I have learned so much from: Alexander Medin, Lino Miele, Petri Räisänen, Juha Javainen, Bert Yogson, Sri K. Pattabhi Jois, Sharath Rangaswamy, David Swenson, John Scott, Igor Odriozola, Ron Reid, Marc Darby, Bill Brundell, Danny Paradise, Jonas Rådahl, Ratheesh Mani, Gustav Björkman, Lasse Nyberg, and Rolf Naujokat.

Thank you for sharing your skills and for your guidance during times when I have been a little lost in my yoga practice.

Chapter 1: What is Yoga?

No one knows exactly how old yoga is. The oldest archeological evidence of yoga's existence are some stone carvings portraying figures in different yoga poses that were found in the Indus Valley, on the border between Pakistan and India. The findings are estimated to come from around 3000 BCE Yoga was first mentioned in the Vedas, a collection of writings from around 2500 BCE.

CLASSICAL YOGA IS BASED ON THE EIGHT LIMBS THAT Patanjali wrote down in aphoristic form in his Yoga Sutras, 200 CE. His writings are based on the Vedas, whose knowledge had been transmitted orally from guru to student, until they were written down. The Yoga Sutras consist of 195 aphorisms, 196 in some editions. In these, Patanjali systemized yoga and gave it a philosophical form. The Yoga Sutras are divided into four books, or chapters, called pada. They are: Samadhi Pada, which describes what yoga is; Sadhana Pada, which gives instructions on how to practice yoga; Vibhuti Pada, which mentions obstacles that might occur in the pursuit of yoga; and Kaivalya Pada, which describes liberation from obstacles that create imbalances in life. In Sadhana Pada, Patanjali describes the eight limbs: Yama, Niyama, Asana, Pranayama, Pratyahara, Dharana, Dhyana, and Samadhi.

Yama—Self-restraints

The first limb, Yama, is about self-control and describes five moral codes that describe how to live a worthy life and how to interact with our surroundings. Ahimsa—do not hurt anyone, including yourself; Satya—commit to truthfulness; Asteve—do not steal; Brahmacharya—live humbly and act in moderation; Aparigraha—do not be greedy. Do not expect to receive anything back when you give, that will keep your mind pure.

Niyama—Inner Observances

Gives guidelines on how to treat yourself with respect and how to create good habits. Shaucha—purity, both on the inside and on the outside. Santosha—contentment for what we have and don't have. Tapas—doing just enough,

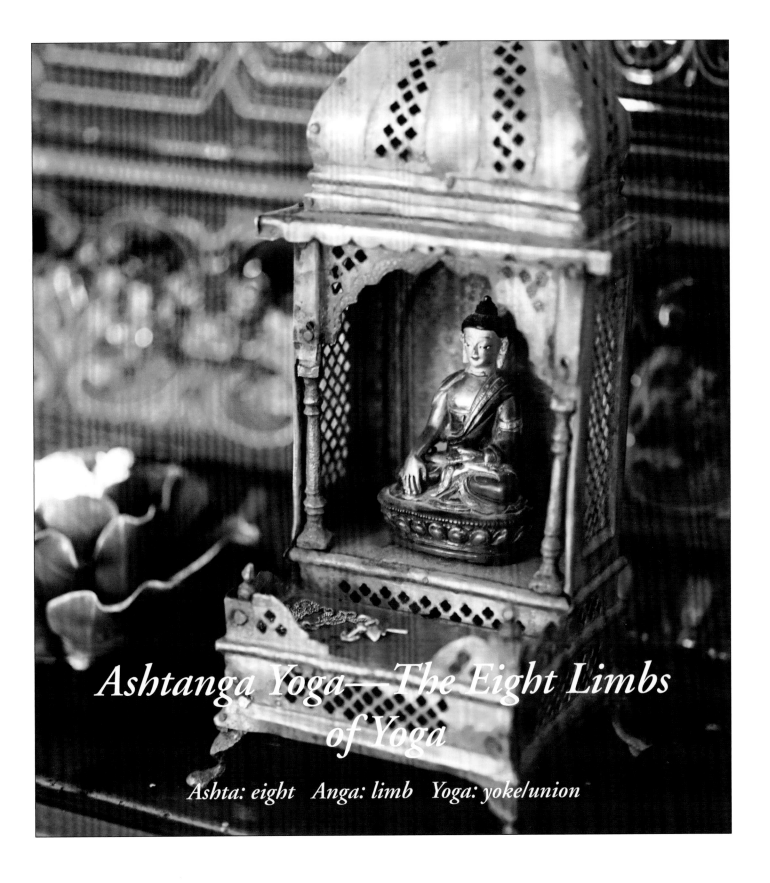

Ashtanga Yoga—The Eight Limbs of Yoga

Ashta: eight   Anga: limb   Yoga: yoke/union

whether sleeping, eating, exercising, working or relaxing, and the body and mind will be purified. Svadhyaya—self-analysis; Ishvara pranidhana—be humble before a higher intelligence or God to let go of ego.

Asanas—Movements

The only one of the eight limbs that has anything to do with yoga movements. In ashtanga vinyasa yoga they strengthen, cleanse, and soften the body and mind. The breath links the movements. Practicing the ashtanga vinyasa yoga series will prepare you to face the challenges in life.

Pranayama—Breathing Exercise

Pranayama is a method to regulate and optimize the energy flow in the body.

Pratyahara—Withdrawal of the Senses

The first step towards shifting the focus to your internal world. Here you practice your ability to control and withdraw your senses from external objects. The goal is to shift the focus from the external world and turn inwards to get to know your inner self.

Dharana—Concentration

Here you practice concentration and the ability to control and focus the mind. Dharana is the first step towards achieving deep meditation.

Dhyana—Meditation

A meditative state, where you leave your ego and achieve a deep connection to the present moment and your inner self. Only then can you truly connect to your surroundings.

Samadhi

The final goal of yoga. A state of utter stillness transcending the body and mind, where the life force flows freely and you achieve a connection with the Divine and the rest of the world.

Yoga as a Tool

Yoga is not a religion, but more like a science of life. It is the oldest system in the world for personal development, where it is important to put equal focus on the body, mind, and soul. Yoga means yoke/union: uniting the individual self (jiva) with the divine consciousness (Brahman).

Simply put, we will find the answers we are looking for within ourselves—we are all like uncut diamonds—we are all God and yoga is a tool to find ourselves again, since most of us seem to get lost after our birth. We are essentially born pure, but our experiences, paths, and actions do not always stem from our inner divine, and we need to reconnect to that truthful inner being inside of us.

It is easy to get the impression that you must follow a strict diet, learn all about yoga philosophy, and change your life drastically if you want to begin practicing yoga. But yoga can fit into any lifestyle, we can embrace it no matter where we are or what lives we are living. I believe that the biggest challenge is to fit yoga in to your daily life where work, children, partners, family, and friends already fill our busy schedules.

You can read plenty of books on yoga, you can learn Sanskrit, or interpret Patanjali's Yoga Sutras—you might even learn his writings verbatim and repeat them in Sanskrit, but if it doesn't manifest itself in you, what is the effect? Preferably, you should practice meditation and yoga every day, so that it is nurtured inside of you. It won't happen just by reading about it, but you need to let it grow and manifest itself by the act of doing it. Be patient, it won't happen right away, but if you are persistent and pay attention, yoga will teach you to understand your body's signals. All you need to do is listen instead of taking it for granted.

Yoga is a philosophical system that includes ethical rules and attitudes—such as being kind to yourself and to other living beings, and other practical tips and methods that makes life easier and more harmonious and healthy. When the mind and body are in harmony with

HOW YOGA AFFECTS YOUR BODY

- Yoga strengthens and stretches the muscles.
- Yoga counteracts physical tensions and softens stiff muscles.
- Yoga improves the blood circulation in the entire body.
- The body's ability to take up oxygen increases and in turn you feel more alert and your energy increases so that you have the ability to do more.
- Yoga teaches your body to relax when needed, and it is a powerful tool to counteract stress.

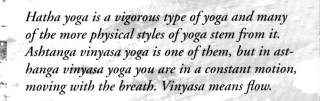

Hatha yoga is a vigorous type of yoga and many of the more physical styles of yoga stem from it. Ashtanga vinyasa yoga is one of them, but in asthanga vinyasa yoga you are in a constant motion, moving with the breath. Vinyasa means flow.

What is yoga?

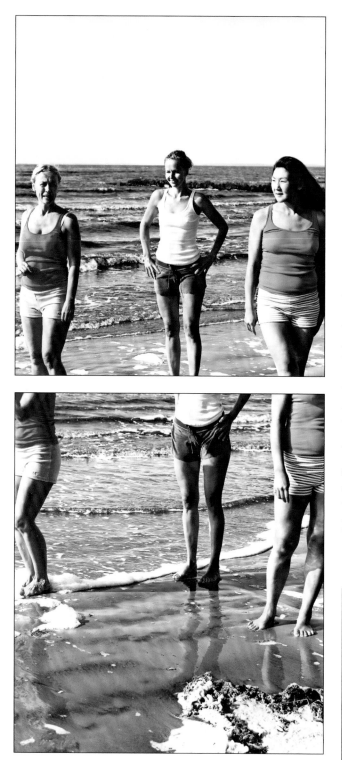

each other, a desire to maintain a healthy lifestyle follows naturally. Slowly but surely yoga increases each individual's potential. For many of us, our first encounter with yoga will be like falling in love because we'll feel the positive effects of our practice almost right away. Maybe you'll start to sleep better and deeper, or feel less affected by stress. All of a sudden you will notice the positive changes that yoga brings into your life.

A lot of it has to do with allowing yourself time for yoga. As women we have a tendency to take care of everything else before we take care of ourselves, and we tend to push things intended for us forward for a later date, but in yoga you will face yourself and stay present. Begin by finding a place and opportunity where you won't be interrupted. Roll out your mat and breathe.

A regular yoga practice will make you more flexible, which in the long run may remove back pain, stiffness, depression, and simultaneously improve your self-esteem. Your body will get strong and flexible, like a temple where you can age with grace.

So why not try it out and see how it will make you feel? Give yoga a few weeks of your life. After a while it just becomes something that you do as part of your life. Something that makes you feel better.

The exercises in the book stem from hatha yoga, but because I practice ashtanga vinyasa yoga daily, the postures are colored by my experience and practice. There are many different styles of yoga and none is more beautiful or better than the other. You simply have to try different styles until you find one that suits you.

The spine consists of thirty-three separate bones that are called vertebra. Together they make up a column that protects the delicate spine that is an essential part of the central nervous system and whose function is to send information from the brain to the body and back again. Through yoga the spine becomes more flexible; in China, a flexible spine is considered a guarantee to a long life.

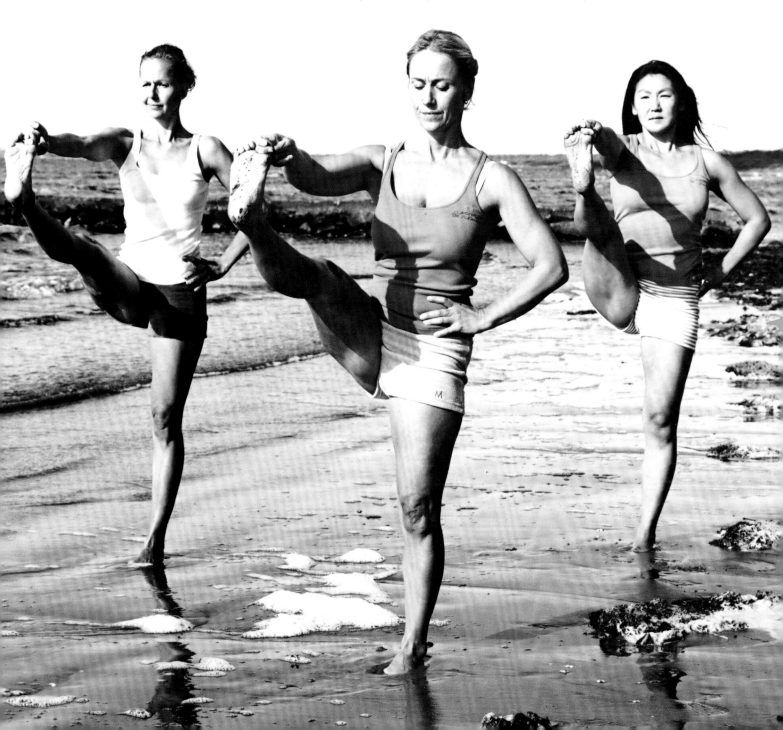

Do your practice and all is coming.
—*Sri K. Pattabhi Jois, the founder of ashtanga vinyasa yoga*

Chapter 2: The Breath— Learn to Stay Present

According to an old Indian saying we are only allowed a certain amount of breaths in a lifetime. That means that if we learn how to lengthen each breath, we can live longer. It is also said that we do not use our entire lung capacity when breathing. It's pretty exciting to explore what could happen if we actually used more of it! Who knows—perhaps we would become wrinkle-free, happier, and smarter. I believe that there are only positive things to add to the list if we learn how to consciously use our breath to full capacity.

BREATH IS LIFE. BREATH WILL infuse your yoga practice with life when you breathe deep and consciously in each pose, so that your practice becomes dynamic. Let the breath join the movements. Feel like you move with the breath in a flow. In the long run, your breath will lead your movements.

The yogic breath begins with a deep inhale that continues to move through the chest all the way up to the collarbones. Most of us use shallow breathing high up in the chest. That sometimes causes us to lift our shoulders or draw our stomachs in as we breathe in. We can only pick up a fraction of oxygen when breathing this way, but we have the ability to breathe much deeper. By using yogic breathing, you will learn to do that and feel better in the long run. You will learn to breathe through the nose with the mouth closed, and to inhale and exhale to full capacity, so that your lungs are completely filled and emptied even when you move through the poses. Full breaths use the diaphragm to massage the internal organs and the heart.

The Diaphragm

The diaphragm is our most important breath muscle. We use it when breathing into the abdomen area. When we inhale the diaphragm contracts as the chest expands,

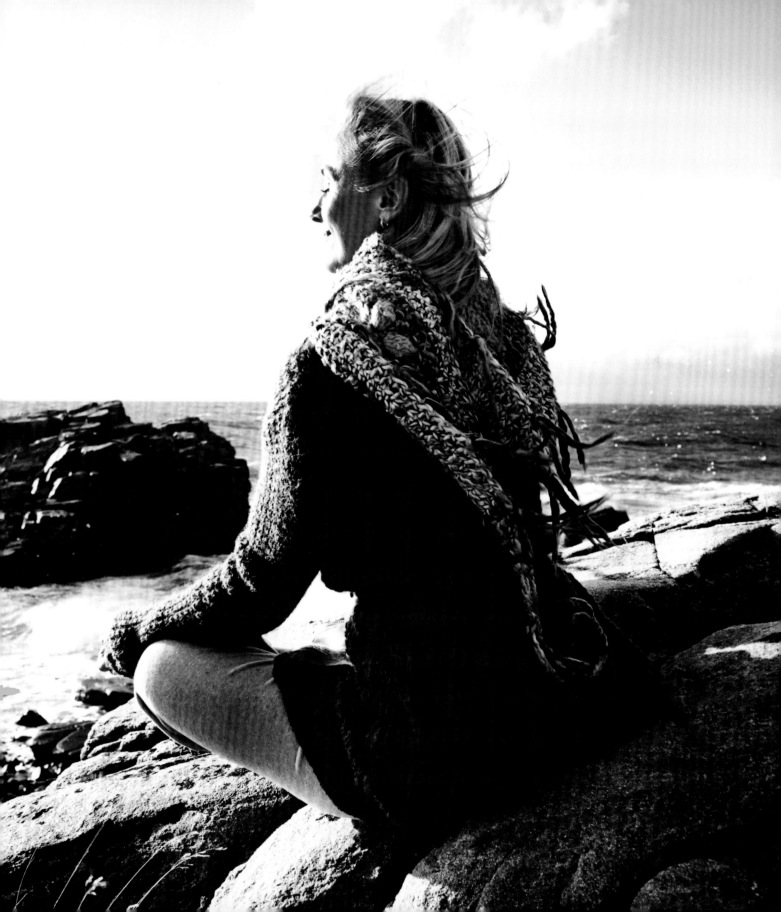

and it works sort of like a wall between the chest cavity and the abdominal cavity. When the muscle is activated, it is pulled down and the volume of the chest cavity increases, which creates pressure under the chest cavity. The lungs expand and fill with air. When the diaphragm relaxes the pressure decreases and the air exits the lungs.

Take a Deep Breath

The breath can teach us how to control our emotions. There is a reason why you encourage a stressed or angry person to take a deep breath. That extra breath can relieve a fit of rage and calm someone that is stressed out, and it can even ease pain. Usually when in pain, we tend to hold our breath instead of doing the right thing—to breathe. To let the breath flow freely and consciously through the body can soothe menstruation aches. The breath is also an excellent tool during pregnancy and during childbirth.

The yogic breath will soon affect your regular, natural breathing and you will notice that you no longer get out of breath when you hold a speech, ask your boss for a raise, or when you do other things that normally would stress you out and make you nervous. Your calm breathing will become a part of your personality: you will become more grounded and calm for each deep breath that you take.

Breathing Exercise

Sit comfortably right on the sit bones either against a wall or on a chair, and relax. Relax the lumbar spine and release the pelvis towards the floor. Mindfully extend the spine all the way from the tailbone to the tip of your head. Slightly tuck your chin towards your chest without loosening the neck. Close your eyes, or focus your gaze on a neutral point. If you notice that you are rounding your back, or if your legs start to hurt, just lie down and keep breathing.

Natural Breathing

Start out by allowing your breaths to roam freely through your body, just like you normally breathe. Keep the mouth closed and breathe through your nose as naturally as you allow your thoughts and feelings to come and go without paying attention to them. Notice your breath. How is it today? Observe your breath without judging it. Feel how it pulsates through your body like a wave that rises up against a sandy beach, soft and organic. Note that there is a slight pause after each exhale. Feel how your spine extends, and your chest rises without drawing up your shoulders. Imagine that you are opening up your heart to the sky. Feel the relaxation in the shoulders. Feel the space between your ears and your shoulders increase. Let all the tiny face muscles relax. Release the jaw and keep the mouth soft. Let it rest like a little smile on your lips. Feel the gaze behind your eyelids, steady and turned down. The eyelids are resting softly over the eyeballs. Feel how the forehead is completely free of tension and the space between the eyebrows is soft. Sit like this for 4–5 minutes before you go into conscious breathing, where the goal will be to deepen each inhale and exhale.

Conscious Breathing

Now you have surpassed the normal breathing to a more conscious breathing where each inhale and exhale is deeper. Now you breathe all the way down to your belly. Imagine that you release unnecessary emotions on each exhale. It could be feelings of achievement, stress, anger, or perhaps sorrow. Whatever it may be, you don't need those feelings at the moment. Imagine that you clear the lungs on each exhale and create room for the inhale—the new, the hope that fills you. Allow your body to follow the breath. Feel your chest expanding on each inhale and feel it sinking on each exhale. If your thoughts are distracting, try focusing on your breath on each inhale and exhale.

I'm inhaling
I'm exhaling
I'm inhaling
I'm exhaling
I'm inhaling
And so on…

Focus on the breath and resist the body's signals that tell you "my hand is itchy," "my foot has fallen asleep," or "I need to change this position"—learn to listen to your body so that you can determine if you really do need to scratch your nose or change your position. In turn, the body will learn to rest with your thoughts. All the little brain ghosts will calm down and the breath will become a tool to cultivate peace. That's what we want to achieve. That's when the moment with your breath will become meditative and you can sit completely still and stay present in your breath—a place where we as stressed westerners have such a hard time to find, but that we long for. We always feel like we have so much to do before we can actually sit down and just breathe.

The Victorious Breath

Once you have achieved conscious breathing you can conquer a more forceful breathing technique, ujjayi pranayama, which means the victorious breath.

Continue to breathe through both nostrils while keeping the mouth closed. Direct your breath towards the back of your throat, where your larynx is. Tone the muscles at the back of your throat so that the breath canal becomes a smaller ventilation tube. When you breathe this way your breath will become audible from the back of the throat, and not from the nose. You pull the breath in through the nose, but as far back into the throat as possible. There, behind the collarbones, imagine a little room. In that little room you let the breath beat against the walls so that a hissing sound is heard.

Place your hands on your chest and feel how the chest expands during each inhale, and how it sinks on each exhale. Place your hands under your armpits without crossing your arms in front of your chest, and feel how the chest expands. Feel how you fill your body with breath on each inhale. Place your hands on your lower back and feel how you breathe into it. You can also place your palms over your ears and listen to your breath.

Imagine that you breathe deeply through your body all the way down to the pelvis and back up through your belly and chest until the breath exits your throat on the exhale.

BENEFITS OF THE BREATH

- Calms the mind and you learn to cultivate focus.
- The breath fills the body with energy and gives the poses the power they need.
- The breath will make the yoga poses meditative.
- Proper breathing will increase the oxygen in the blood, which stimulates the blood circulation in the entire body.
- A powerful and controlled breath purifies the larynx, the air passages, and the lungs, and it clarifies the voice.
- Ujjayi breathing can be strengthening and calming for the nervous system, and it aids the digestion and removes phlegm. Sickness is caused by excess of mucus, air, and bile according to ancient yoga scriptures.

Why Do We Breathe with our Mouths Closed?

When you use the powerful ujjayi breathing with your mouth closed, you are building heat in the body and the air stays longer in the airway's mucous membrane, which is full of blood vessels. The air has time to heat up, and the nose cilia cleanse the air that is going into the lung. When you exhale, an opposite effect occurs. The exiting air moistens and heats the mucous membrane in the nose, which means that the body maintains proper heat and moisture levels.

Imagine that each inhale fills our bodies with new power and life. With each exhale we release the old: sorrows, stress, achievement pressure, or anger. Without judging the breath simply notice if the inhales or exhales are longer. Then the breath becomes psychological. Is it easier for you to lengthen your exhale, than it is to lengthen the inhale? Perhaps it is easier for you to let go of the old than it is to receive the new? Or maybe you have a difficult time with lengthening the exhale? Perhaps you like to hold on to the old, and have a hard time of letting go. Sometimes this will vary. I find it very interesting to listen to my own breath. It never lies. If you are happy and excited, your breath will be quicker and more enlivened.

The Body Remembers

According to yoga philosophy the body has a sensory memory and everything that you have done and experienced with it, is stored inside of it. The body never forgets anything. By practicing yoga, you give your body and mind an opportunity to move on and leave old experiences behind you.

When I was 22 years old I did something called rebirthing. That means that I used my breath to be reborn. It is just one of the many alternative therapies that I have tried out through the years. My mother always said that I was such an easy child to give birth to (I'm the third child), so I was never scared to try rebirt-

hing when Rosen Method Bodywork therapist and yoga teacher, Anna Rinnman, suggested that I try it with her. We were breathing, sort of hyperventilating, and after a while I stopped breathing completely and Anna had to bring me back to life.

After a few times Anna suggested that I obtain my birth records. She said that mothers usually forget or repress childbirth. I did as she suggested and I was surprised at the answer: I was close to death when I was born. I had Petidin in my bloodstream, which made me passive during the delivery. The umbilical cord had wrapped itself around my neck in two loops. When I came out I was blue and I was sucking on mucus.

My mother had repressed my birth, perhaps because it was such an unpleasant experience, or maybe because she was affected by Petidin as well. The importance of this story is that my mother's story was entirely different from what actually happened, but when I tried rebirthing my body remembered it, because you cannot trick the body. I believe that things are stored in the body—even before we have mastered the words to express our feelings. The breath helped me to connect with emotions that I had stored and still store in my body, so that I could begin to understand them and embrace them even when unpleasant.

If you are not used to breathing exercises, take it easy at first. Allow it time—let it take the time that you need. Your experience does not need to be like mine. Your experience of yoga and the breath will be unique because you are unique. Today I am able to take deep and long breaths, and I have mastered breathing techniques that are powerful and that require that you retain your breath for a long time. But it took me a long time and I still practice every day. In the beginning I almost had feelings of anxiety when I practiced the breathing exercises. I believe that those emotions were connected to my difficult birth. It took me a long time to get over those feelings, but I didn't stop trying out of fear; instead I saw the breathing exercises as a challenge. I believe in the power of thought—if you visualize that you will be able to do yogic breathing exercises one day, it will work out that way.

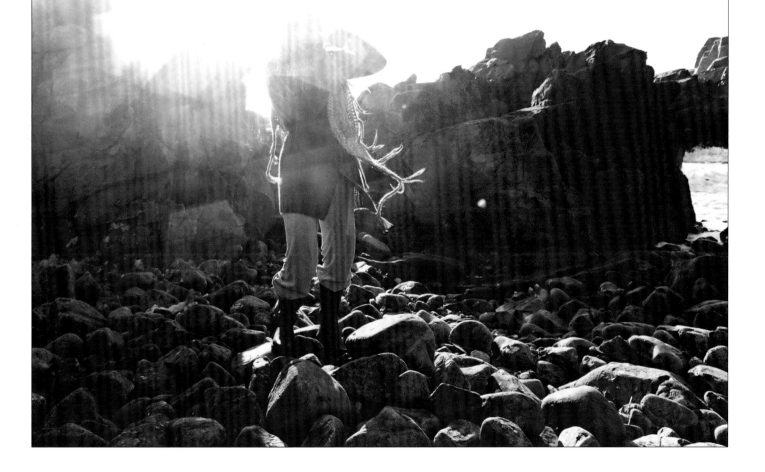

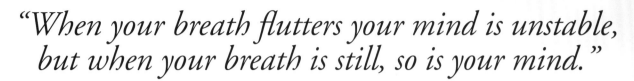

"When your breath flutters your mind is unstable,
but when your breath is still, so is your mind."

Hatha Yoga Pradipika
Swami Swatmarama 1350–1400

Chapter 3: Bandhas, The Body's Energy Locks

Susanne Lanefeldt was quite right in the eighties when she encouraged all women to engage the perineum with all their might on TV. All women can benefit from stronger pelvic floor muscles. I would like to pass the torch on from Susanne to all women and urge you to practice the pelvic floor exercise daily, and engage in it for your own sake.

IN YOGA WE USE CERTAIN ENERGY

Mula Bandha—The Root Lock
Activate Mula Bandha:

Sit in a comfortable cross-legged position. Begin by localizing the sphincter at the anus and holding it in and simultaneously draw it up. Make sure that you don't tense up the butt muscles but that you try to isolate the movement to the sphincter. Imagine that you activate the muscles around the urethra upwards and continue the movement up and into the body.

Uddiyana Bandha—The Diaphragm/ Navel Lock

Uddiyana means to lift up and that is exactly what you do. Uddiyana bandha is located about two fingers beneath the navel and when you activate it, you are pulling in and lifting the lower abdomen. You are carefully pulling that point up on an angle, and back towards the spine to support the lower back. Imagine it as if you have an inner corset, an inner power center behind the navel where mula bandha and uddiyana bandha meet.

It is not unusual when emotions come up to the surface when you do yoga, because you are releasing different tensions in the body. Don't get frightened, you have always carried those feelings so it is nothing new. Sometimes you will feel very happy during your yoga practice, or a little sad or annoyed. Don't let these feelings distract you, but stay in the pose and keep breathing. Yoga is something you have to master every day.

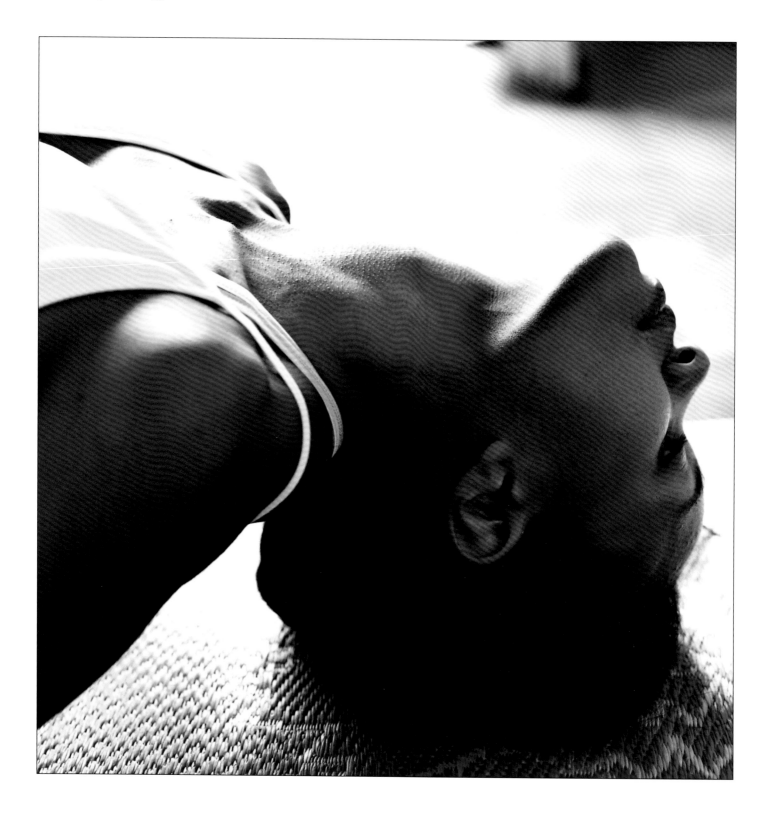

Activate Uddiyana Bandha:

Place two or three fingers below the navel (horizontally) to find uddiyana bandha. Your point will be right below the bottom finger. When you activate your energy locks, do it in a soft flow. The contractions roll the pelvis forward and lengthen the tailbone downward so that the lumbar spine is protected in the exercises. When you activate uddiyana bandha in a motion, the power comes from inside and not from the muscles of your back.

Jalandhara Bandha—The Throat Lock

If the root lock lengthens the spine upward, the throat lock is what opens up and supports the upper back and the head. It protects the neck in all of the backbends, and it keeps the head balanced right on top of the vertebral column, as opposed to having it hanging slightly in front.

Activate Jalandhara Bandha:

Sit in a cross-legged position. Engage the navel in and up to ground your pelvis. Then lift the chest. It should feel like the movement comes from inside, like you are lifting the breastbone.

Draw the chin slightly in without losing the entire neck. Relax the neck muscles and pull the shoulder blades down.

You may feel stiff in this position at first, but be patient, with training it will feel natural. The throat/neck lock helps the head to balance right over your heart so that the weight is taken off the neck as the mind and thoughts are calmed. The back is stretching simultaneously as the movement and pose helps you to lead with your heart, as opposed to leading with your head, which can flex the spine instead of flexing at the hips.

Use The Locks

Use the locks in your yoga when you practice the asanas, or poses, to help the body to find the most optimal position and to protect the vertebrae so they are not pulled together too forcefully in flexion or extension. How much you should engage the locks depends on the pose. By activating the locks you facilitate the muscular structure to help the body stay upright, which relieves the body from pressure. It might not feel like that in the beginning but have patience and it will get easier with time.

When we first learn how to use the energy locks we need to pay a lot of attention to engage them and at the same time relax other muscles, but with time it becomes second nature.

Strive to engage mula bandha and uddiyana bandha in all the poses and they will be more effective. Jalandhara bandha is mostly used during breathing exercises.

Chapter 4: Sun Salutations— Begin Your Day by Saluting The Sun

Just like the name suggests, sun salutations are a salute to the sun and a beautiful way to begin the day. I can guarantee you that already after the first sun salutation you will find some sort of inner peace. Sun salutations have been used for thousands of years to strengthen, warm up, and purify the body and mind. The sun salutations appear in some of the world's oldest scriptures, the Yajur Veda and the Rg Veda. You can practice the sun salutations every day to warm up, soften, and prepare the body for the day ahead. The early morning is the best time to practice yoga, while the sun is rising and the stomach and the mind are empty. No matter what poses you choose to do from this book, you can always begin your practice with the sun salutations. You can do as many as you like, but in ashtanga vinyasa yoga you usually do five sun salutations A and five sun salutations B.

Sun salutations as shown by yoga teacher

Viveka Blom Nygren, 41 years old

"I began practicing prenatal yoga in 1990, then I had a big break from it before I took up ashtanga vinyasa yoga in 2000. I saw the transformation in my good friends who had just begun practicing yoga and it made me want to start as well. Yoga has changed my life. You can actually divide my life into "before" and "after" sections. Since I started practicing yoga, I feel connected to myself, and in turn I am living the life I want to live. To me yoga is like a guiding star that I can turn to for energy for both my career and for my everyday life. Yoga makes me happier, calmer, and more balanced."

Sun Salutation A
Surya namaskar A

The starting point for all standing poses and the sun salutations is Samastitihi. Stand upright with both feet firmly on the ground with arms hanging by your sides and the back straight—this is perhaps the hardest of all poses. Feel how you are standing. Are you using the entire foot, or are you leaning to one side of the foot? Maybe you are leaning to one hip when you stand "straight up." Are you letting go of the stomach and over-arching the lumbar? When you begin practicing yoga you will become more conscious of your body. How you are standing. How you walk. How you use your body. Instead of taking the body for granted you will ask yourself: How does this feel? Why do I have a headache or a backache? How do you use your feet, your roots, your foundation? Think about how it feels. Yoga is all about listening to your body.

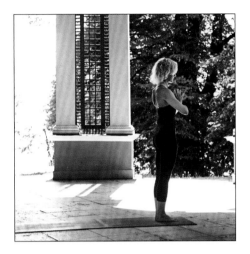

1 Pranamasana

Bring palms together in front of your chest and collect yourself.

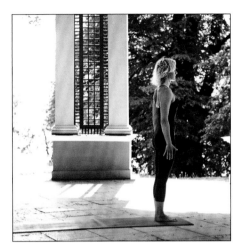

2 Samasthiti

Release the hands by your sides.

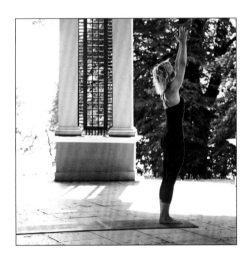

3 Utthita Tadasana

On the inhale: Reach your arms up above the head without lifting your shoulders. Feel as if you are extending up to lengthen the spine. Your gaze follows the hand. Bring palms together over your head.

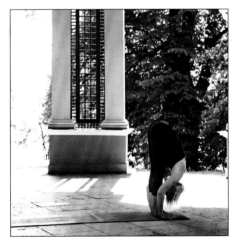

4 Uttanasana

On the exhale: Fold your torso over your legs, the bend happens at the hips. Place the palms by your feet. Relax your neck and press the tip of your nose against your legs. If you can't reach the floor with your hands, bend your knees and lean your chest against your thighs. Set it as a goal to eventually straighten your legs.

Salutation A

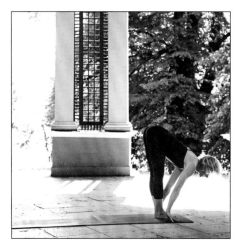

5 Lengthen Your Spine

On the inhale: Lengthen the spine, draw your shoulders back. Imagine that you are stretching out the spine from the tailbone all the way to the head. Place the hands as far down as possible.

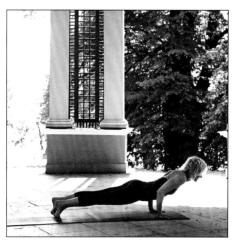

6 Chaturanga Dandasana

On the exhale: Press the palms against the ground and jump back. Place the feet hip-distance apart and lower your entire body until your arms are at a 90 degree angle. Keep the elbows as close to your body as possible.

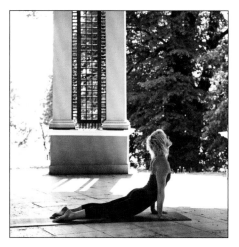

7 Urdhva Mukha Svanasana

On the inhale: Come up into upward facing dog by shifting your body forward and pressing the palms down, while the toes un-tuck. Press the tops of the feet into the ground, stretch the arms and open up your chest and try to extend your back into a backbend. Move shoulders back and down.

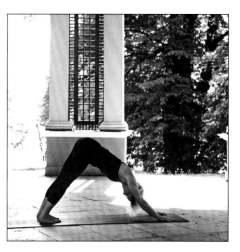

8 Adho Mukha Svanasana

On the exhale: Come into downward facing dog and stay here for 5 breaths. Press the palms into the ground and spread the fingers. Hands are shoulder-width apart and the feet hip-distance apart. Try to reach the heels toward the ground. Lengthen the space between your shoulders and ears by imagining that you are lengthening the spine without arching your low back.

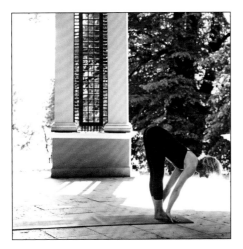

9 Lengthen the Spine

On the inhale: Press the palms down into the floor, jump the feet forward in between the hands, and lengthen your spine. Eventually you will be able to land on straight legs.

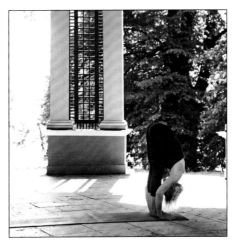

10 Uttanasana

On the exhale: Fold forward from the hips, press the tip of the nose against your legs, and relax the neck.

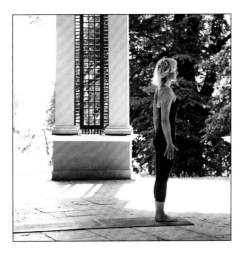

11 Samasthiti

Release the hands by your sides.

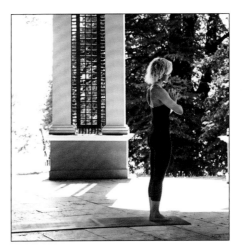

12 Pranamasana

Bring palms together in front of your chest and collect yourself.

Sun Salutation B
Surya Namaskar B

Sun salutation B shown by yoga teacher

Cecilia Wikner, 39 years old

"I started practicing yoga over ten years ago. I was very curious about yoga and what it was. I began by practicing a very calm style of yoga and then I practiced prenatal yoga during my first pregnancy, but it wasn't until we moved abroad in 2000 that I began regular yoga practice. That's when I tried ashtanga vinyasa yoga for the first time and it felt as if I had found home. Yoga makes me happy. It gives me an incredible energy and calms me simultaneously. It is a fantastic combination. Yoga is so much more than what you do on your mat. I try to cultivate it in my daily life by doing simple things such as to take a deep breath, relax, and roll my shoulders back—yes, that actually helps me during stressful moments."

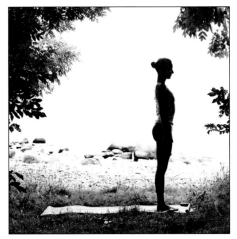

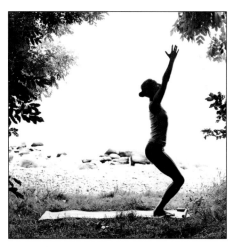

1 Samasthiti

Release the hands by your sides.

2 Utkatasana

On the inhale: Bend your knees and sink your hips low with heels pressing into the ground. Reach the arms up over your head, but sink your shoulders down. Follow the hands with your gaze. Bring palms together over your head.

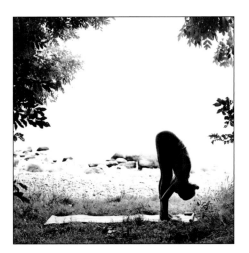

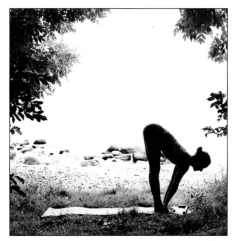

3 Uttanasana

On the exhale: Fold torso forward, initiate the bend at the hips. Place the palms by your feet. If you don't reach the floor, bend your knees and rest your chest on your thighs. Relax your neck and press the tip of the nose against the legs.

4 Lengthen the Spine

On the inhale: Open up the chest and pull shoulders back. Imagine that you are lengthening the spine from the tip of the tailbone all the way to the head. If possible, try to place your palms flat on the floor.

Sun salutation B

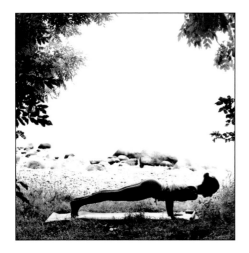

5 Chaturanga Dandasana

On the exhale: Press the palms down into the floor and jump your feet back. Keep the feet hip-distance apart and lower the entire body towards the ground until your elbows are at a 90 degree angle and you are in a low push-up position. Keep the elbows close to your body.

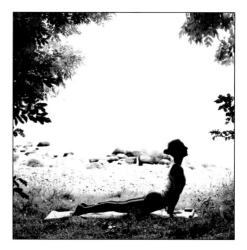

6 Urdhva Mukha Svanasana

On the inhale: Come into upward facing dog by shifting your body forward on your arms, and roll your toes over so that the tops of the feet are pressing into the floor. Stretch the arms straight, and open up the chest and try to backbend in your upper back. Draw shoulders back and down.

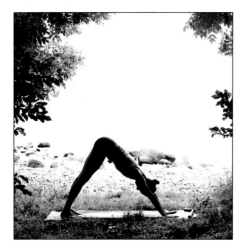

7 Adho Mukha Svanasana

On the exhale: Come into downward facing dog. Press your palms into the floor and spread your fingers wide. The hands are parallel and shoulder-width apart and the feet are hip-distance apart. Spin your left heel towards the right foot onto the ground. Step your right foot forward between your hands, closer to the right thumb.

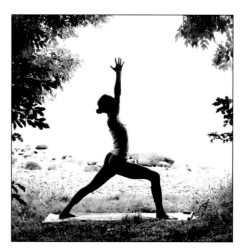

8 Virabhadrasana

On the inhale: Bend your right knee into a 90 degree angle and reach arms up. Bring palms together over your head and look up at your thumbs.

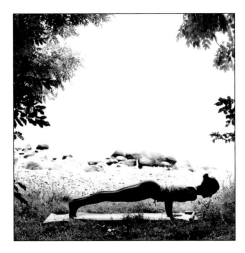

9 Chaturanga Dandasana

On the exhale: Place hands by the sides of your right foot. Step the right foot back so that it is parallel with the left foot and hip distance apart. Lower down into a low plank position.

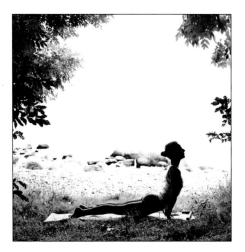

10 Urdhva Mukha Svanasana

On the inhale: Come into upward facing dog by shifting your body forward onto your arms, and roll over toes so that the tops of the feet are pressing into the ground. Straighten arms, open up the chest and create a back-bend in your upper back. Draw the shoulders back and down.

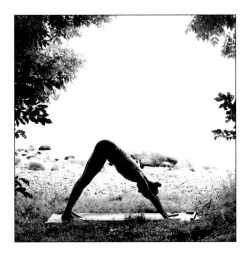

11 Adho Mukha Svanasana

On the exhale: Come into downward facing dog and spin your right heel towards your left foot.

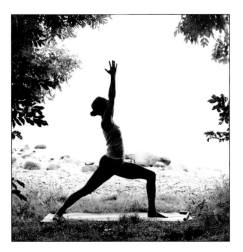

12 Virabhadrasana

On the inhale: The left foot steps forward in between your hands, closer to the left thumb. Bend left knee into a 90 degrees angle and reach your arms up. Bring palms together over your head and look up at your thumbs.

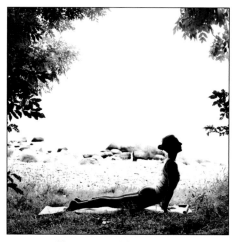

13 Chaturanga Dandasana

On the exhale: Place hands by the sides of the left foot. Step left foot back and lower down into a low push-up position.

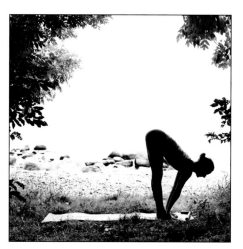

14 Urdhva Mukha Svanasana

On the inhale: Come into upward facing dog by shifting body forward onto the arms. Roll over your toes so that the tops of the feet press down into the ground. Stretch the arms, open up the chest and try to bend your back backwards like a bow. Draw the shoulders back and down.

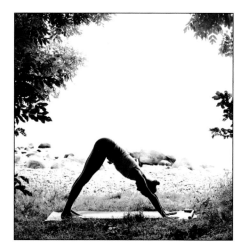

15 Adho Mukha Svanasana

On the exhale: Come into downward facing dog and stay here for 5 breaths. Press the palms into the floor and spread your fingers. Place the hands shoulder-width apart and the feet hip-distance apart. Work on trying to reach the heels towards the floor. Lengthen the space between your shoulders and your ears and imagine that you are stretching out your spine without overextending (curving) the lower back.

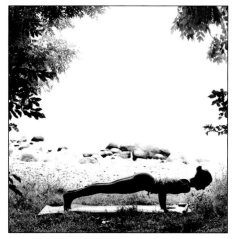

16 Lengthen the Spine

Press the palms down into the floor and jump your feet in between your hands on the inhale, and stretch your back. Eventually, you will be able to jump and land with legs straight as you press the palms down.

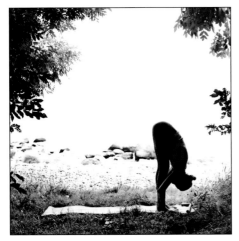

17 Uttanasana

On the exhale: Fold torso forward over your legs and press the tip of the nose against the legs and relax the neck.

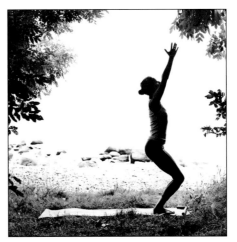

18 Utkatasana

On the inhale: Bend the knees, stretch the arms up to the sky. Bring palms together and gaze at your thumbs.

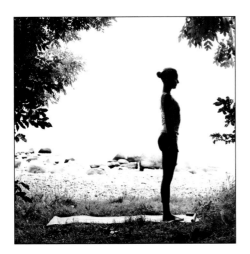

19 Samasthiti

Let the hands fall to the sides of your body.

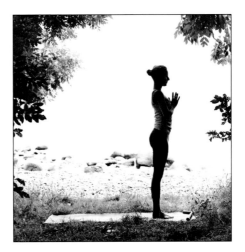

20 Pranamasana

Bring palms together in front of your chest and collect yourself.

Chapter 5: Menstruation Issues and the Days Before Your Period

To most women, the worst time of the month is during the first days of their period or the days leading up to it. The mood is not at its best and the tummy is aching. It can be anything from a dull pain to an excruciating pain that leaves you bedridden. Some women even feel nauseous as part of the deal. There is help. Some yoga poses alleviate menstrual pains, but results demand that you do the poses on a regular basis, at least a few times a week.

THE BREATH IS PART OF THE FOUNDATION IN YOGA: The breath improves the blood circulation in your body and therefore your muscles get more oxygen. When we breathe deeply, our bodies are able to relax, which facilitates blood circulation and the body's ability to pick up oxygen. When we stop our breath, or when we use shallow breathing, the body locks itself and pain arises. When we are hurting, we tend to strangle the breathing, but if you breathe into the pain instead, it will relieve the pain. That is my experience during menstrual pains.

The yoga poses and the breath facilitate in relaxing us, and when we are relaxed, the pain eases.

You should do the exercises on a regular basis to achieve the best results, four to five times a week for about 10–15 minutes is a good amount. Don't put pressure on yourself, just follow the instructions carefully and try to keep the times. And first and foremost—be humble to yourself.

TO RELIEVE HEAVY BLEEDING

Press fresh lemon juice into cold or warm water and drink to cleanse your system. Lemon cleanses the blood and increases the body's ability to get rid of toxins, which improves digestion and strengthens the immune system. Lemons also have an astringent effect that can keep the bleeding in check, if you have issues with a heavy flow.

TO ALLEVIATE PAIN AND SWELLING

Brew a cup of weak peppermint tea by using 0.4 ounces of peppermint and adding two cups of water. Add lemon juice from one lemon. Peppermint is antispasmodic and it aids digestion and alleviates flatulence. In addition, it is mildly stimulating and relieves menstruation.

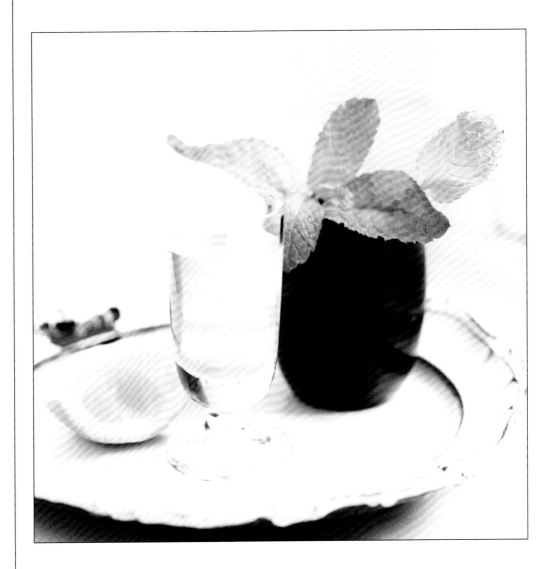

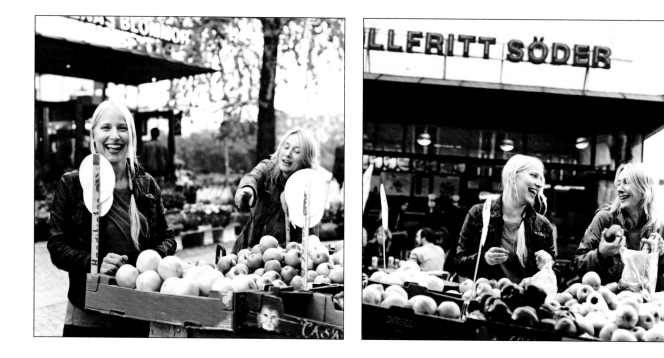

Allow the Body to Rest

During menstruation and pregnancy, loosening of the pelvis requires that the body rests. Allow yourself to rest and to not do the poses fully during the first few days of menstruation. To achieve best results:

• Breathe! The breath is the most important part of yoga. Breathe deeply in through the nose and out through the nose.
• Wear comfortable clothes.
• Do this sequence four to five times a week.
• Take it easy during the first few days of your menstruation cycle.
• Don't eat or drink an hour before or after these exercises to avoid energy being wasted on digestion.

A regular yoga practice can alleviate the menstruation pains in the long run but it will also give us time to go

Studies show that every third woman is suffering from menstruation cramps, and every tenth woman has such severe problems that she becomes bedridden during her menstruation. According to a study conducted at the University of Luleå, physical activities soothe the pains connected to menstruation. Young women suffer the most from menstrual pains, but the aches usually disappear after the first pregnancy.

inwards and not stress, like we so often do as women when we hurry to get everything done. Before and during the menstruation cycle, we enter an entirely different state. Our hectic lifestyles don't allow us to rest, not even during menstruation. Yoga will connect you to your body and you will feel more balanced in your life.

The yoga poses shown by yoga teacher

Hilda Norberg, 30 years old

"I found yoga in the Dales in 1997. That was my very first time trying out yoga. I've become more focused and approach things in a new way since I started practicing yoga. Yoga has connected me to my own body in a new way, and my posture has improved. The journey has been tough, but it has been well worth it. I have learned a lot that I would have been unaware of otherwise."

Supta Baddha Konasana—Reclined Bound Angle Pose/ Butterfly

BENEFITS

This is a great preventative pose for menstruation issues. It opens up the groin and allows the lumbar to rest, the areas that usually hurt during menstruation pains.

HOW TO DO IT

- Lie on your back on the floor or a yoga mat, and support your back with a bolster or a pillow.
- Bring soles of the feet together so that knees are pointing out to the sides—like the wings of a butterfly.
- Stay in this pose for 3–10 minutes and breathe, preferably using your ujjayi breathing.

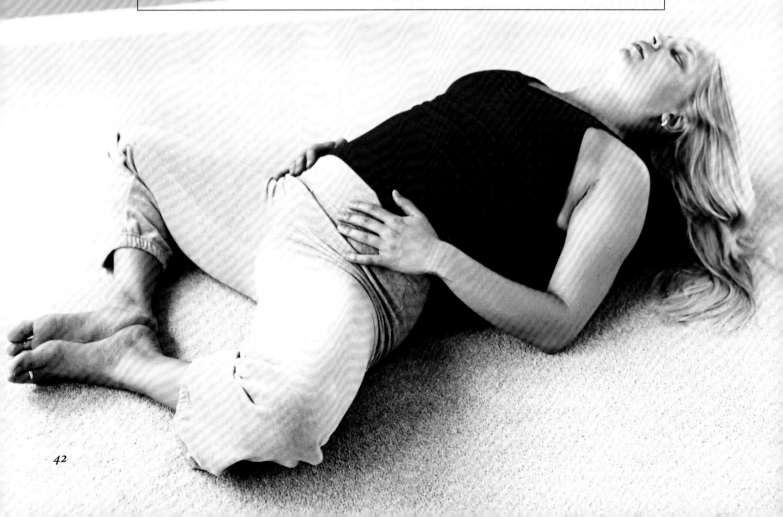

Frog Pose

BENEFITS
This pose has the same effects on the body as Supta Baddha Konasana. It improves the blood circulation and opens up the hips and groins.

HOW TO DO IT
Sit with legs underneath you, knees pointing out to the sides and toes pointing in towards each other like a butterfly, but instead of leaning back lean forward, preferably onto a bolster of pillow to support your torso. Lie like this and breathe for 3–10 minutes.

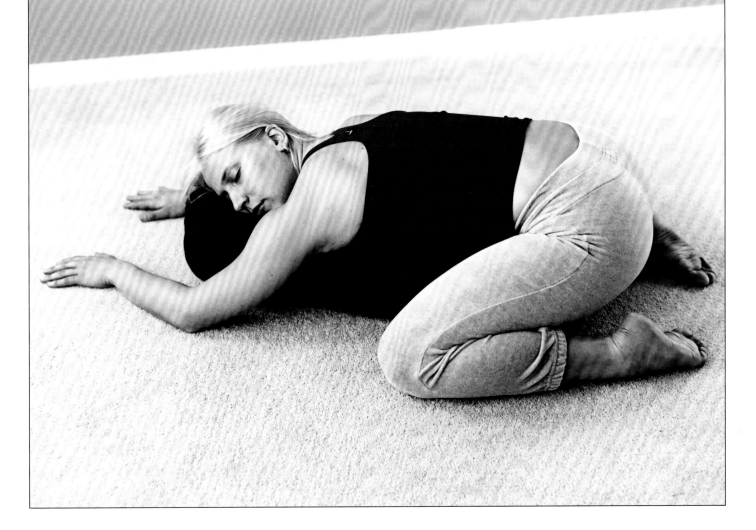

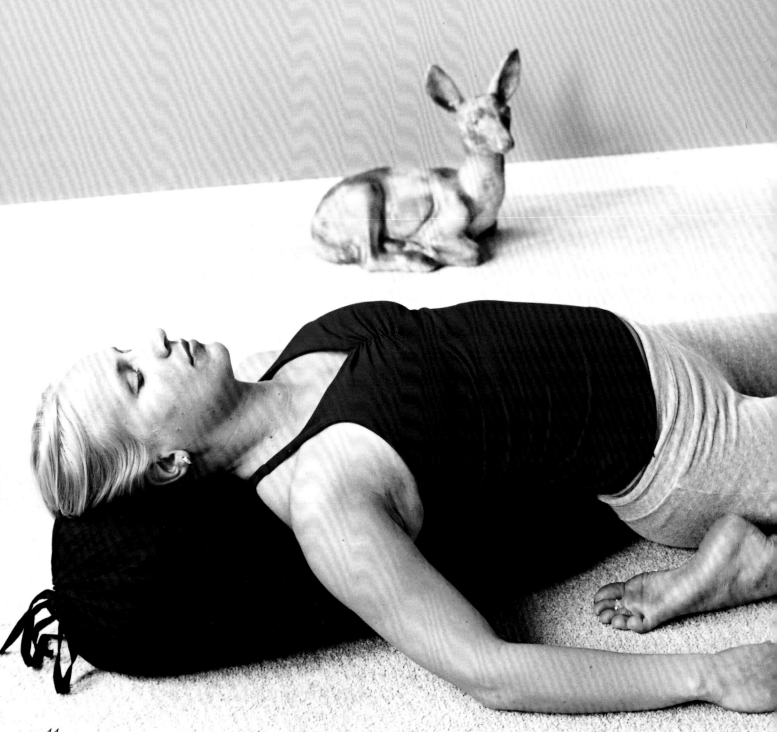

Supta Virasana

BENEFITS
Many women have issues with their bowel movements during menstruation. This pose aids the digestion, blood circulation, and energizes the legs, that tend to feel heavy during the period.

HOW TO DO IT
- Sit down with your shins alongside the outside of your thighs. Toes are pointing behind you.
- Recline onto your back. Support the lumbar and the back with a bolster or pillow.
- Stay like this for at least 25 deep breaths.

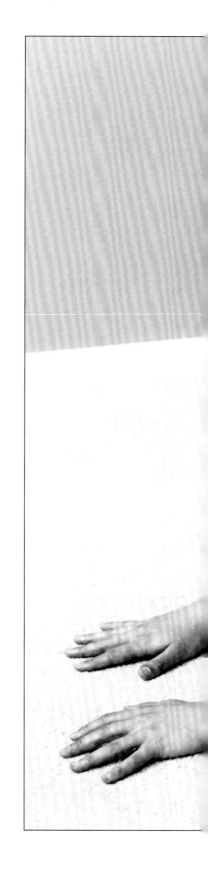

Virasana—Forward

BENEFITS

This is a restorative pose that lengthens the lumbar spine. It releases tension in the gluteus muscles, where a lot of tension accumulates during menstruation. All poses are calming to your mind, but this particular posture can really help you connect to what is inside of you. Another name for it is child's pose and it is reflective and easy to relax in.

HOW TO DO IT

- Begin by sitting on your knees.
- Fold torso forward and let the forehead come to the ground. Try to keep your buttocks against your heels.
- Stay in this pose for at least 25 breaths.

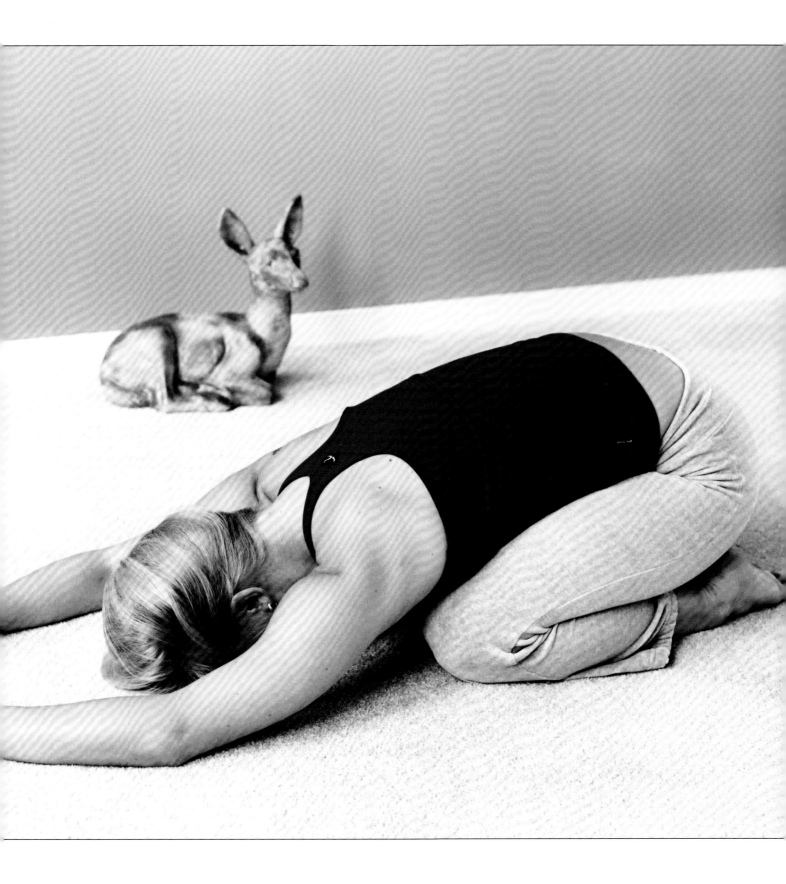

Menstruation Issues

Baddha Konasana – Bound Angle Pose/Seated Butterfly

BENEFITS
This pose is said to stimulate and strengthen the entire pelvic region. It also stimulates the heart and is good for blood circulation.

HOW TO DO IT
- Sit with the soles of the feet together in front of you. You can use a wall to make sure that you are sitting up straight. Press down the outside of the thighs towards the ground.
- Breathe deeply in this pose for 3–4 minutes.

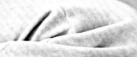

Baddha Konasana against the wall

BENEFITS
The same as in sitting baddha konasanama, but here you relieve the legs from supporting weight, as they often swell during menstruation.

HOW TO DO IT
- Lie on the floor against a wall.
- Move the buttocks as close as possible to the wall. Swing legs up against the wall, but keep the butt on the floor. Rest the soles of the feet against each other, knees pointing out to the sides. Rest hands on the stomach or on the legs.
- Lie like this for 15–20 breaths.

Chapter 6: The Young Woman in Her 20s–30s

These are years when there are a lot of things happening in a woman's life during a short time. Perhaps you are studying and feel stressed before exams or schoolwork in general. Perhaps you have a job that demands a lot from you, and you spend a lot of time working. The career pressure from other people is especially tough on a woman without any children, but perhaps your own expectations are the toughest ones?

PERHAPS YOU FEEL AS IF YOU ARE IN A RUSH. These years can be very stressful and full of expectations. By the age of thirty, you are expected to have a good job with good chances for a career, and you may feel you should have a life partner that you have begun discussing children with.

Live in the Present

To many of us this is the time when we are hunting for a better life, but might not feel as good in the present. That is exactly why—because life is spinning by way too quickly—you need to pause during this age, to find peace of mind, and moments to rest your mind and recharge. For some strange reason it always seems like many young people are in a hurry, like they are about to miss a train.

Stress

We are not talking about a life that is running on a low jet but on a major welding flame. But, if you learn to take one day at a time you have everything to gain. Studies show that young women often feel stressed out and that they put high expectations on themselves to be good at many things. Taking it easy is something you can learn and yoga is a good tool to use to find calm and ease within yourself when it feels like the world is spinning out of control.

We have different ways of handling stress. While one person might be handling stress pretty well, another one might be completely destroyed by it. A tiny bit of stress might even be stimulating, but prolonged stress can cause psychological and physical damage.

Give yourself 10 minutes of yoga, two or three days a week, and I promise that your days will be easier to handle.

The yoga poses are shown by yoga teacher

Johanna Ljunggren, 33 years old

"I found yoga when I was expecting my daughter Vera. When I began practicing yoga I connected to parts of myself that I had forgotten about, or repressed. I realized that to feel whole, I needed to get to know all parts of me. We are like big puzzles when we are born, all the pieces are there, but the puzzle needs to be put together. We are not always aware of all the pieces. In the beginning we are entirely dependent on others to survive. For each breath that we take, we divide the puzzle pieces to experience life from the outside. Often we lose the ability to see how all the pieces are connected, which is necessary to come back to a state of wholeness again. I believe that anyone can find the connection between the pieces by practicing yoga."

Ardha Rajakapotasana—Hip Opener

BENEFITS

If you sit down a lot, which tends to happen when studying, it is good to stretch out the gluteus muscles, the inside of the thighs, and the groin. This pose strengthens the hips and creates agility in the pelvis, the hips, the seat, and the lumbar.

HOW TO DO IT

• Stretch the left leg behind you. Press the top of the foot into the ground. Point the heel up to the ceiling and keep the entire foot in line with the leg.
• Bend your right knee and try to position the right shin parallel to the front of your mat, so that right knee and right foot are parallel to each other. In the beginning, before the hips are as open, the foot is usually angled more towards the left groin area, instead of in line with the right knee.
• If possible, lean forward and feel the stretch in the hip and the groin. Use your breath to deepen the pose for 5–10 breaths before you switch legs.

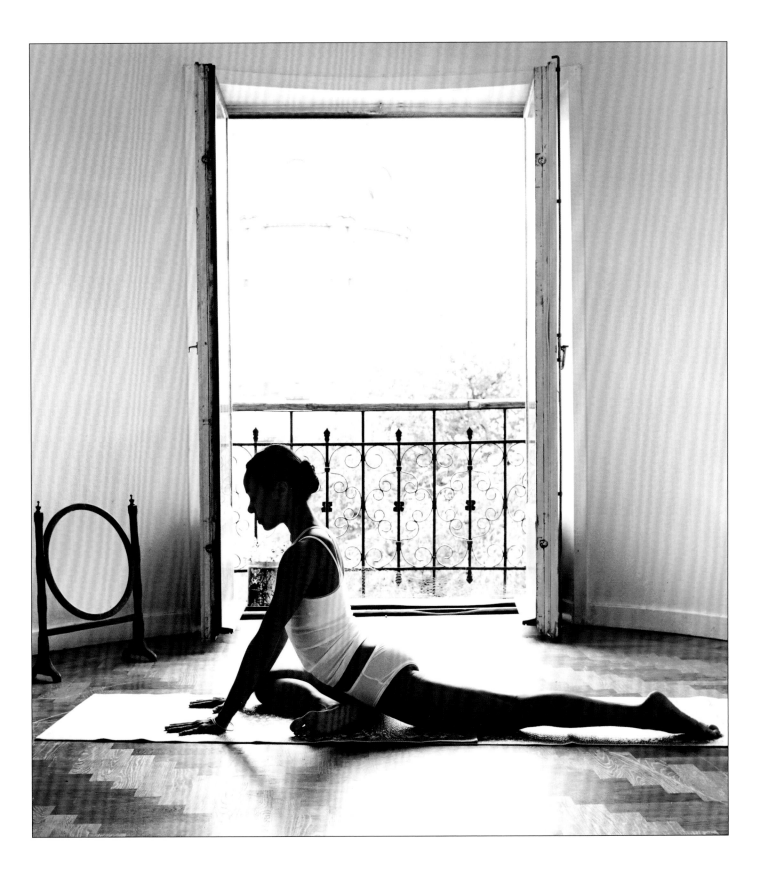

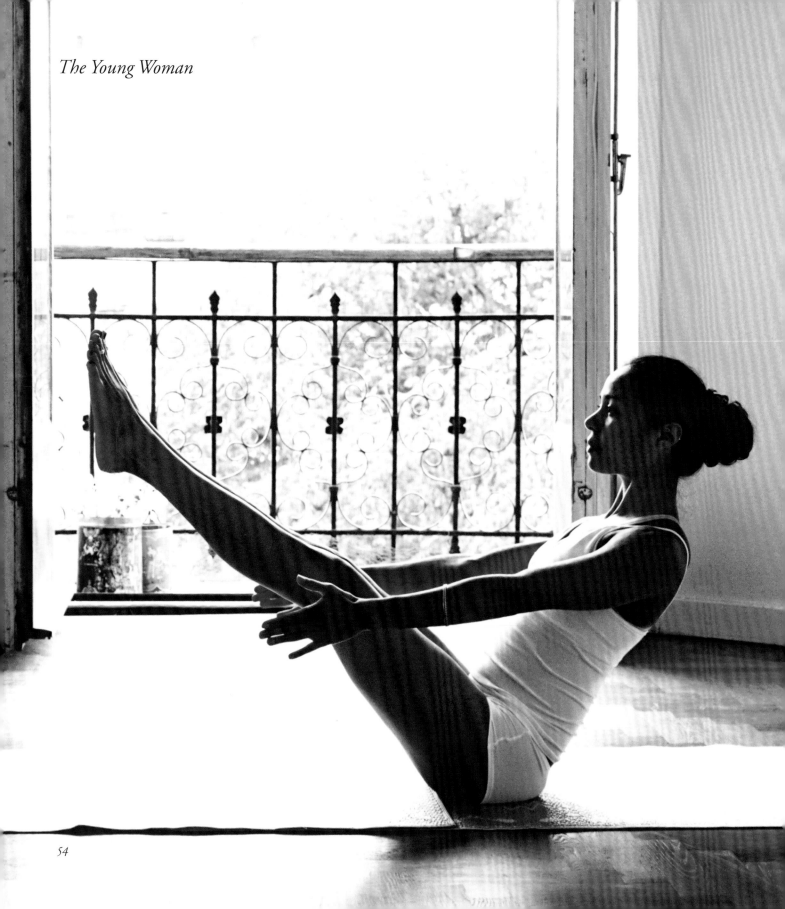

The Young Woman

Navasana—Boat Pose

BENEFITS
This pose strengthens the back, the legs, and the core and it is said to aid digestion and soothe stress.

HOW TO DO IT
- Come into the pose from a seated position.
- Hold the back of the knees and stretch the legs up towards the ceiling, as you stretch your chest up simultaneously.
- Let go of the legs after a while, but don't let straight legs be a priority over a hunched back. The most important thing in this pose is that you maintain a straight back, so if you need to, bend your knees.
- Maintain this pose for 5–10 breaths. Rest and repeat five times.

Spinal Twist

BENEFITS
Tension in the back, the hips, and the shoulders are allevia-ted in this pose. It is a great pose to practice if you've been sitting down for a long time.

HOW TO DO IT
- Lie on your back and take your left knee up to your chest. Then twist the left knee over to your right side.
- Stretch your left arm out to the side in line with the shoulders.
- Turn your head to the left and look over the left shoulder Feel the stretch in your left side. Imagine that you breathe into the tensions to release them whenever you feel a bit of discomfort in your muscles.
- Imagine that you breath moves through every single vertebra and lengthens your spine.
- Stay in this pose for 5–10 breaths, and repeat on other side.

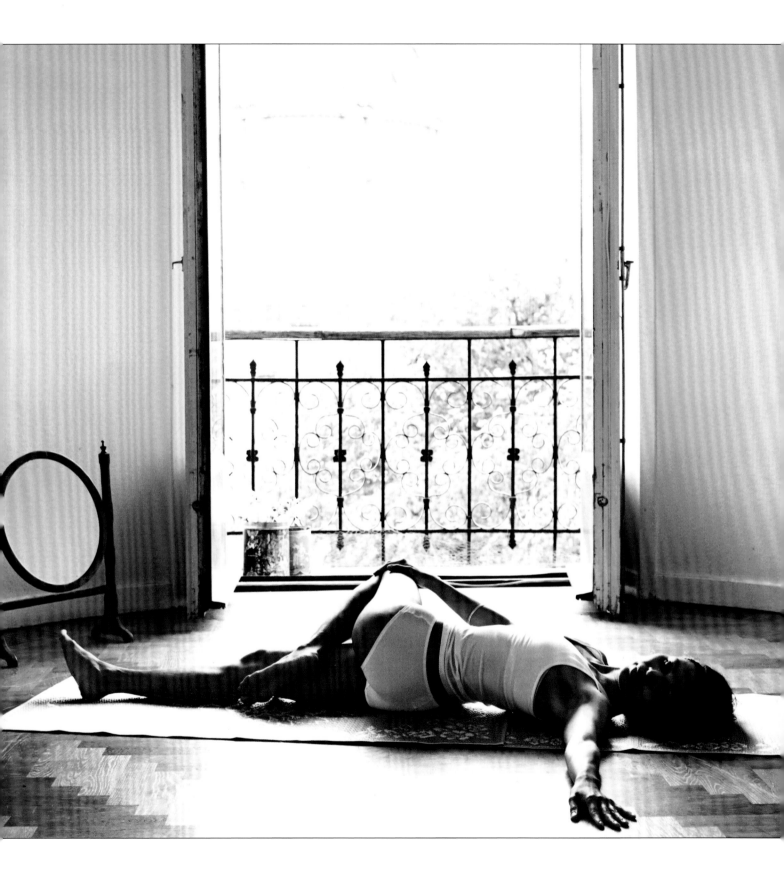

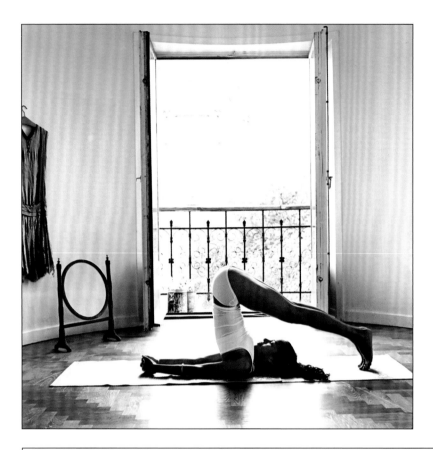

Halasana—Plow Pose

BENEFITS
Said to relieve fatigue, stress, and stress related headaches. Also aids all throat related issues and back problems, and aid sleep at night. Avoid the pose if you have hernias, high blood pressure, sciatica, or if you have a serious back injury.

HOW TO DO IT
• Lie on your back and tuck your knees into your chest. Inhale and lift the legs and the feet a little bit.
• Lift your buttocks with your hands. Stretch the neck. Think of lengthening the space between the chest and the hips, so that you don't round your back.
• Lower the feet and the legs toward the floor, behind the head. In the beginning you can support your back with the hands, and later when you feel strong enough in your neck and the pose feels more comfortable, you can clasp the hands behind your back and try to reach your toes toward the floor.
• Lie like this for a maximum of 10 breaths. Carefully roll down onto your back, vertebra by vertabra. Rest for a moment before you take a fish pose.

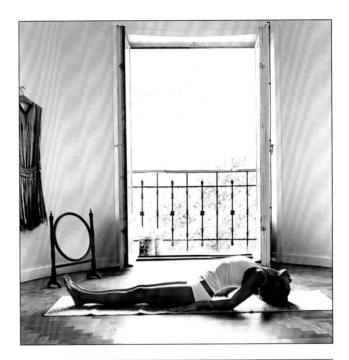

Matsyasana—Fish Pose

BENEFITS

It is good to do a fish pose after the plow pose. This asana increases blood flow to the face and strengthens lung capacity through the opening of the chest. Fish pose is said to aid stomach issues, and to relieve tension in the neck and the shoulders. It is said that in order for us to become emotionally whole we need to open up our chests and minds.

HOW TO DO IT

- Lie on the floor on your back. Keep the legs together and lengthen the ankles down so that the toes point straight ahead.
- Carefully lift yourself onto your elbows, but maintain the buttocks on the floor so that the upper body looks like a bow.
- Lean the top of the head back towards the floor. Lift the chest and feel how it opens up. Be mindful of where your shoulders are. Try to increase the space between your shoulders and your ears.
- Stay in matsyasana for 10 long breaths and come out of the pose slowly.

If you want to challenge yourself in the pose, you can place your hands in your lap so that you no longer support yourself on your elbows. Or you could bring the palms together in front of your chest. Then slowly come down with your neck and shoulders toward the floor, and bring the knees toward the chest and hug them with your arms to stretch out the back. Use your breath to calmly and slowly take yourself out of this movement.

Gomukhasana—Cow Face Pose

BENEFITS

When we sit down a lot, our shoulders and the upper back tend to get very stiff. This can cause bad posture, but first and foremost block the flow of prana (life force) in the body. This pose relieves the tension and facilitates a free flow of prana. The legs are stretched in this pose and the ankles get more flexible. Gomukhasana is also said to stimulate the will and inner power.

HOW TO DO IT

- Sit down and cross your legs in front of you so that the knees are on top of each other. Bend the right foot towards your left hip, and your left foot towards the right hip. You can also sit on your knees to modify.
- Keep your back straight and stretch your right arm behind your back, and bend your left elbow toward the ceiling and reach your left hand behind your back until you are able to clasp the hands together. You can use a strap, or a scarf to grab onto if your hands do not reach each other.
- Stay in this pose for 5–10 breaths and pull the left arm up to open up the chest even more. Switch the crossing of the arms and legs and repeat the pose on the opposite side.

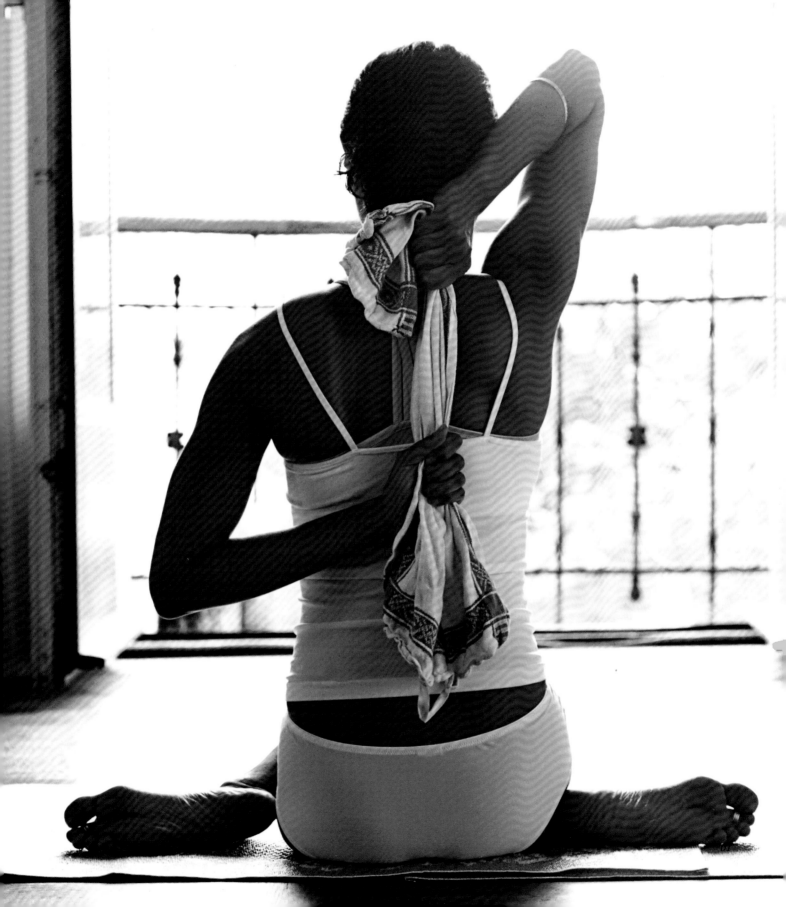

Savasana—Corpse Pose

BENEFITS

Even though this might look like the easiest pose of all the yoga asanas, it is perhaps the most difficult one for us westerners to do. The body is supposed to relax, and at the same time your mind is awake. Staying in this resting pose for 5–10 minutes allows your body to recharge and energize.

HOW TO DO IT

- Lie on your back and have your legs slightly apart and your arms resting along the sides of your body.
- Let the hands rest on the floor with the palms facing the ceiling. Close the eyes and keep your attention inwards.
- To find a sense of calm in the body in this pose, you can listen to a relaxation tape or calming music. Or go through each body part in your mind and feel how it relaxes and surrenders to gravity. Start with the toes and work yourself up to the head, body part by body part.

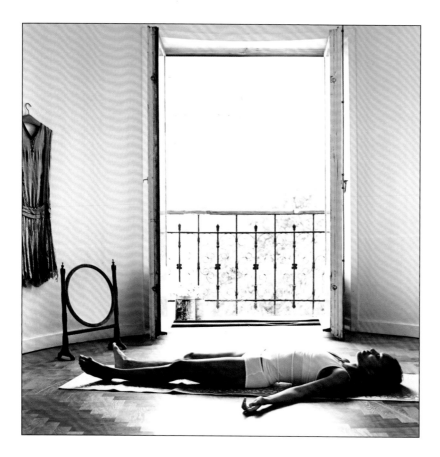

SALAD WITH ORANGES, PUMPKIN SEEDS, AND CHOPPED & SOAKED ALMONDS

Soak almonds (preferably organic) for 24 hours. Slice two oranges and mix with a handful of chopped almonds and a handful of pumpkin seeds. Almonds aid digestion and breathing, and they alleviate inflammation in the body. They are rich in fats, zinc, potassium, B-vitamins, and magnesium, and they have high protein content.

Pumpkin seeds are said to reduce the effects of stress. They contain high amounts of zinc, iron, potassium, B-vitamins, and proteins that enhance the brain's functions. Oranges (vitamin C), strengthen the immune system and shorten colds and other viruses. They reduce cholesterol and keep our skeleton, teeth, and genitals healthy.

Today, there are a lot of discussions about a lack of rest being worse than mental and physical stress. Mental stress is said to increase muscle tension. So even if you don't have a physically challenging job, your risk to accumulate tension in your neck and shoulders is higher if you just "run" and don't learn to listen to the signs of your body. Let yoga help you to pause, instead of taking a smoke break.

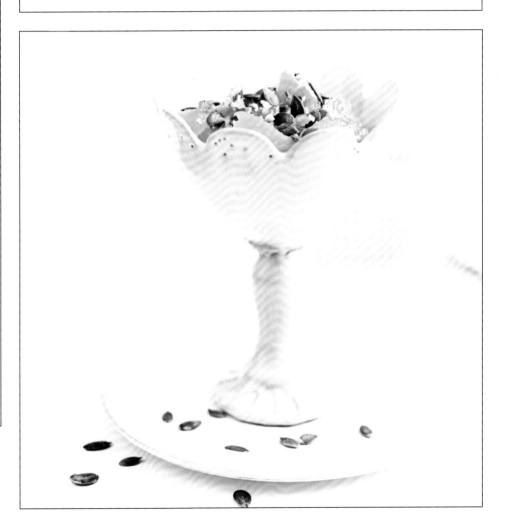

Chapter 7: Pregnancy and After Childbirth

You are about to become a mother. Your body is growing. Perhaps you have always been in a hurry and never quite taken the time to listen to your body. During pregnancy you are no longer capable of hurrying through life. That is the point, so your steps need to slow down.

PRATCING YOGA IS A GREAT WAY to prepare yourself physically, mentally, and emotionally for pregnancy, childbirth, and parenthood. Make use of this time, get to know yourself inside, and cultivate body awareness and strength as you learn to control your breath. Yoga will teach you how to stay present—and you'll need that when you become a mother. You will learn how to not react blindly, but to act with consideration.

To become a mom is such a personal experience, I cannot define it for you. Midwives and doctors will keep track of your health and how fast the fetus is growing, so that is taken care of for you. By practicing yoga, you can build an inner balance and strength that will help you with the big challenges. No matter if you are used to exercising or not, you will benefit greatly and find joy in yoga while getting ready for motherhood.

Yoga poses shown by yoga teacher

Sofia Norén, 31 years old

"In 1997 while I lived in New York, I was looking for an alternative way to stay in shape without getting injured, something that wasn't dance or aerobics. That's when I discovered yoga. To me, yoga is a tool to a deeper connection beyond the physical. The deeper I delve into yoga and myself, the more space I create. I always feel like a beginner in my meeting with yoga and I get even more humble before it every year. Yoga is a friend for life, it never ceases to surprise me and to guide me onto new paths in life."

Sun Salutations for Pregnant Women

Sun salutations are a great way to warm up even when you are pregnant, but the sequencing is slightly different. You can do as many sun salutations as you please. The most important thing is that it feels good when you do it, but four to five of them gets the energy and the circulation going in the body.

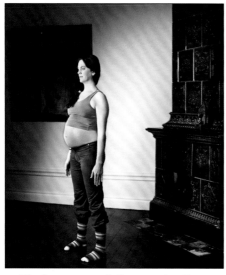

1 Tadasana—Mountain Pose

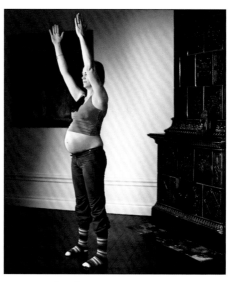

2 Reach the Arms Up

Stand with your feet hip-distance apart and parallel. Feel the connection to the ground beneath your feet. Toes are pointing slightly in, and spread so that the arches of the feet are lifting. Relax your lumbar spine by drawing in your pelvis—sort of like you are lifting up your child from the underside. Let the arms relax by your sides. Feel how you relax in the shoulders. Lengthen and relax your neck and tuck the chin in slightly towards the chest. Transfer the weight slightly forward so that the gravitation line, ear-shoulder-hip, is in line with the highest point on the top of the foot, pada bandha, the foot-lock.

Reach your arms up and shoulder-width apart above your head but without lifting your shoulders. Lengthen the space between the shoulders and the ears. Look up.

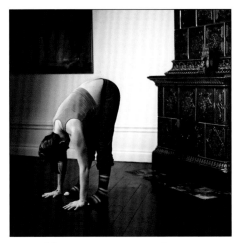

3 Fold Torso Forward

Fold the torso forward and try to touch the floor with your hands. You can bend the knees if you feel any discomfort, or if you can't reach the floor. Relax your neck and lift shoulders up and back.

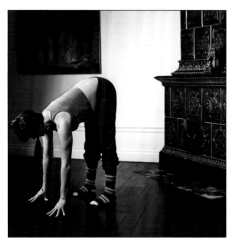

4 Lengthen the Spine

Keep the hands on the ground if possible and lengthen the spine—all the way from the tailbone to the head. Imagine that you are looking between your eyebrows.

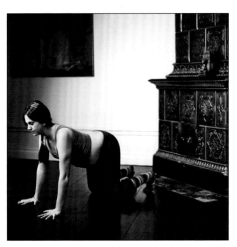

5 Cat Pose

Lower down to your knees and come into cat pose with a neutral spine, without over-arching or rounding the spine. Knees are hip-distance apart and hands are shoulder-width apart.

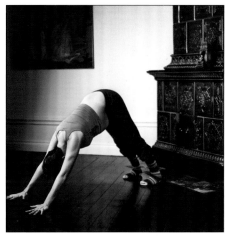

6 Downward Facing Dog

Come into downward facing dog by reaching your hips up. Strive to reach the heels to the ground. The hands are shoulder distance apart. Relax the neck so that it is parallel with the arms and draw the shoulders back. Visualize how you lengthen your spine. Stay here for 5–8 breaths.

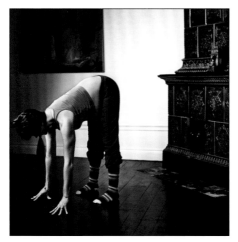

7 Lengthen the Spine

Step out so that feet are hip-distance apart. Leave the hands on the ground if possible and lengthen the legs and the spine from the tailbone to the head. Gaze between your eyebrows.

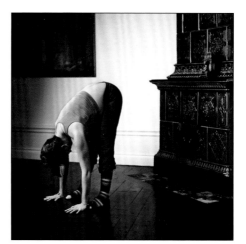

8 Fold Torso Forward

Fold torso over legs as much as possible.

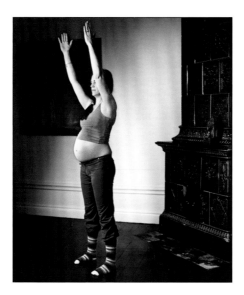

9 Reach Arms Up

Come into standing with arms above the head. If it is difficult for you to stand up with a straight back, bend your knees and support yourself with your hands on your knees, then come up with your knees bent.

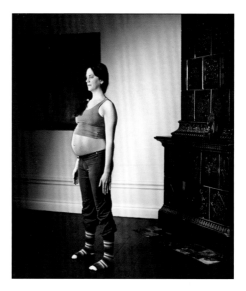

10 Tadasana

Mountain pose—Tadasana

GINGER WATER

If you feel nauseous during your pregnancy or if you have a difficult time with your digestion, try drinking ginger water. Peel an inch or two of a ginger root and cut into pieces. Put into a cup and pour boiling hot water over and let it sit for a few minutes. Add a little bit of honey and squeeze some fresh lemon juice if you wish. Ginger comes from India and is added generously in cooking but also in Ayurveda—a system of medicine from India. The root is recommended during colds, influenza, cough, bad digestion, vomiting, burping, stomachaches, and hemorrhoids. Don't drink too much of it, only one to two cups a day.

"Little one, I welcome your presence into my life, my union with you. When were you not in my life and in my heart?"
—Berber lullaby

When you practice relaxation regularly, you learn to dissolve stress as it occurs. That way you can prevent tensions and exhaustion from building up. You learn to let go, to relax and create opportunities to spend time with the people that are important in your life and with the life that you are carrying inside of you. Pay attention to what is inside of you and get to know yourself and the little human being that you are carrying in your belly by finding your inner calm.

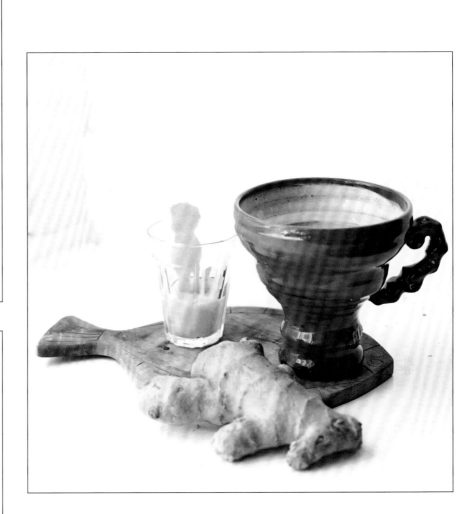

Squatting

Squatting is great for pregnancy, even if it might not be the pose you give birth in.

 We are all different and for some people squatting down without a little stool or a stack of books underneath the buttocks for support works great, while other people need the support to rest the back. If you have varicose veins, hemorrhoids, or feel it in the joints, sit on a little stool to lessen the pressure on the cervix and the pelvic floor. If the legs are swollen and you feel discomfort in this pose, lie down on your back with your legs against a wall and do a squat pose against the wall.

BENEFITS
This pose strengthens the legs, widens the pelvis, and softens the hips. It also aids blood circulation around the belly. The pressure around the abdomen combined with increased circulation prevents constipation, which commonly occurs during pregnancy.

HOW TO DO IT
• Slowly squat down by bending the knees and lowering the pelvic floor towards the ground. Place the feet wide apart and point the toes in the same direction as the knees.
• Gently press the knees wide apart with your elbows and rest the palms against each other or interlace the fingers.
• Lengthen the back and lean forward slightly to relax the backside.
• Maintain this pose and breath with even inhales and exhales for a minute and a half.

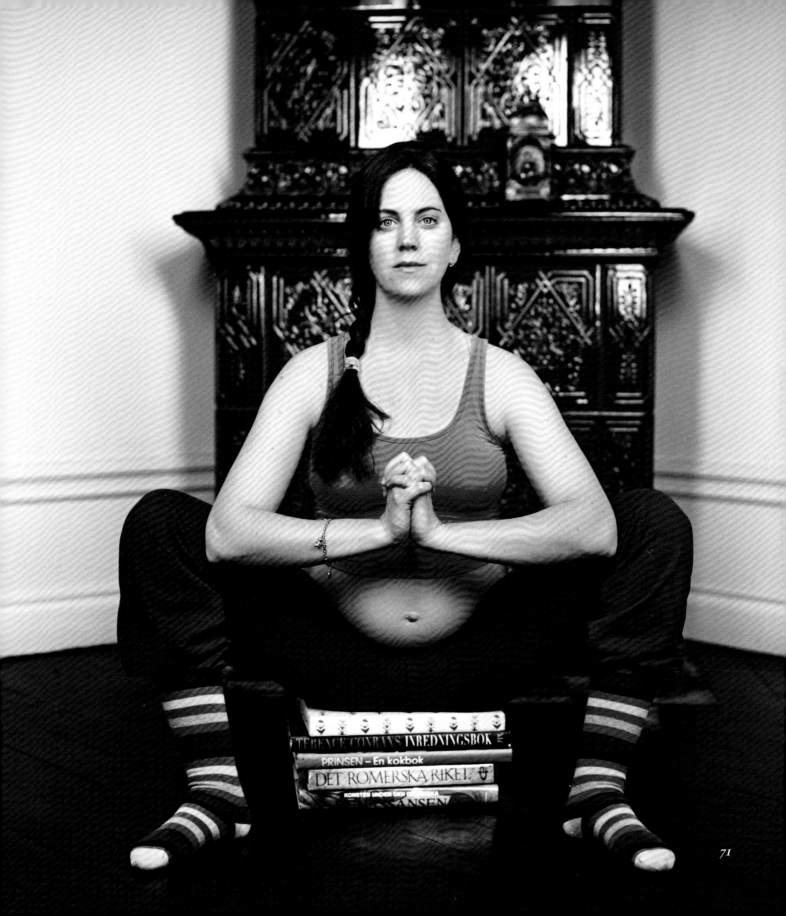

Crossing of the Arms

BENEFITS
Stretches the space between the shoulder blades and relieves tension in the neck and shoulders.

HOW TO DO IT
• Cross the arms in front of your chest. Begin by placing your right elbow over your left elbow crease, then intertwine the arms so that the palms come together. Think of lowering your shoulders so that you don't pull them up to your ears, and try to soften them.

• Gaze towards the fingers and hold this pose as you breathe deeply for a few minutes. Then switch the crossing of the arms. Shoulders, neck, and shoulder blades may feel tender during pregnancy. It almost feels as if the blood is standing still in your veins. The following poses are great during pregnancy but also after childbirth, when you need to soften the shoulders and neck after breast feeding.

Stretching the Neck

BENEFITS
Releases neck and shoulder tension. This pose also lengthens and stretches the spine.

HOW TO DO IT
- Lengthen the spine, all the way to the neck. Gently tilt the chin towards your chest as you lengthen your neck.

- Place hands on the back of your head to stretch the neck. Keep shoulders down and lengthen the space between the shoulders and the ears.

Adho Mukha Virasana—Forward Spine Stretch—Child's Pose

BENEFITS
In this pose your back gets to relax because the baby's weight shifts forward whether you place a pillow underneath your uterus or not. This is a very soothing pose for back pains, which often occur during pregnancy. It quickly alleviates tensions in the lumbar region, or any form of sciatica pains, while it softens the hip joints and pelvic joints and makes them more flexible. The muscles around the abdomen relax and that relieves any stress related contractions.

HOW TO DO IT
• Sit with your legs underneath you and the knees separated out to the sides. The big toes are pointing towards each other and the butt rests on the heels.
• Let the pelvis sink down and get heavy against the feet.
• Relax the lower back and lean forward from the hips. Keep the butt on the heels.
• Stretch the upper body forward and down, and reach the arms in front of you or rest the forehead on the hands. You can stay like this from a few breaths to 3–4 minutes.

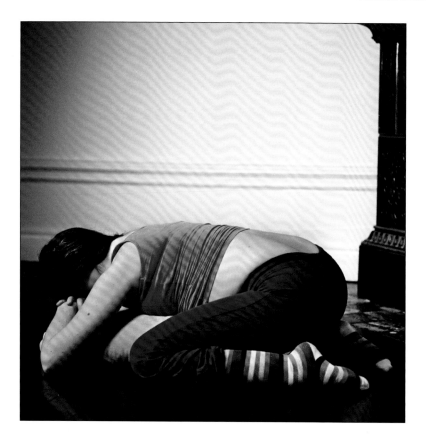

Legs-up-the-Wall Pose

BENEFITS

This pose is both stimulating and relaxing at the same time. It increases the blood circulation in the entire body. During pregnancy we retain a lot of water. Together with the extra body weight it can result in swollen legs and varicose veins. This pose relieves the pressure on the veins and allows the legs to rest. Don't do this pose if you have high blood pressure. You may feel discomfort in this pose towards the end of your pregnancy.

HOW TO DO IT

• Lie down on the back with the legs against the wall. Make sure that your butt is touching the wall and that the torso is straight. Rest your hands on your belly and feel the connection to your baby.

• Lengthen the neck by tilting the neck towards the chest. Relax the back, the head, the neck, and the shoulders. Close your eyes and follow the breath.

• You can lie like this for 3 minutes. Then roll over to one side and rest.

Yoga poses shown by yoga teacher

Sassa Lee, 37 years old, and her daughter Mika

"It took a lot of persuasion on my friend's part to finally convince me to go with her to yoga class. That was in the beginning of 997, and yoga has been a central part of my life ever since. It is difficult to find words to describe what yoga means to me, and all the benefits that came with it, without sounding pretentious. But if I were to mention something, yoga has helped me to cultivate patience, partly through its craft but also because I practice it regularly. Today I have so much more patience with people, in situations and different relationships. Yoga has taught me that it can prove fruitful to not always react to every situation. A reaction is often hasty and requires a lot of unnecessary energy to restore the situation. In the end, everything is the way it should be anyway. The trick is to get there as smoothly as possible."

Pelvic Floor

The pelvic floor is built like a hammock of muscles that attach at the lumbar region and at the abdominal muscles. The muscles stretch straight through the base of the body, from the pubic bone to the tailbone. These muscles need to be strengthened in order to support the uterus and other organs during your pregnancy and after you have given birth.

In yoga you learn to engage energy locks in the body and there are three different ones around the pelvic floor:

Ashwinimudra

Imagine that you are pulling in and up around the anus.

Mula Bandha

Imagine that you are pulling the perineum, the area between your genitals and the anus, up.

Vajroli Mudra

Imagine that you are engaging your clitoris, the area right in front of the urethra, in and up. When you first start out, it will feel as if you are engaging the entire area around your genitals. If you keep practicing, you will learn to localize and isolate engagement in the different locks. Start step by step by breathing in and lifting up each of these areas, and then exhale and release each lock step by step.

Why is it good to train the pelvic floor muscles?

- Increased knowledge and awareness of the pelvic floor muscles can enable you to control the muscles during labor.
- When the pelvic floor muscles are well-trained, the elasticity in the vagina and in the perineum increases, which keeps the pelvis in place. This can affect the inner organs and prevent pressure on the back and the pelvis.
- Your genitals will recover faster after you give birth.
- Pelvic floor training increases the oxygen in the blood, which helps to heal the genitals and recover the muscles faster.
- Prevents incontinence issues, hemorrhoids, and uterine prolapse.
- Your ability to control your pelvic floor muscles might positively affect your sex life.

Pelvic Floor Exercise

HOW TO DO IT

- Begin by identifying the pelvic floor, the area between the tailbone and the pubic bone. You can lie down on your back with your legs bent or sit with your legs crossed. After a while, if you feel discomfort lying on your back, turn so that you are lying on the side instead.
- Breathe naturally. Begin by engaging the sphincter around the rectum. Continue forward and up and around the vagina and the urethra opening, like you are about to lift something up.
- Inhale and engage the muscles. Relax on the exhale. Lie like this for a moment and localize all the little muscles around the pelvis. If you are comfortable you can continue to engage these muscles for a little bit longer.
- Continue to hold on a count to five and then slowly release. Rest in between the contractions if you need to. Repeat 7–10 times.
- Finish off with short and rhythmic engagements of the muscles for as long as is comfortable.

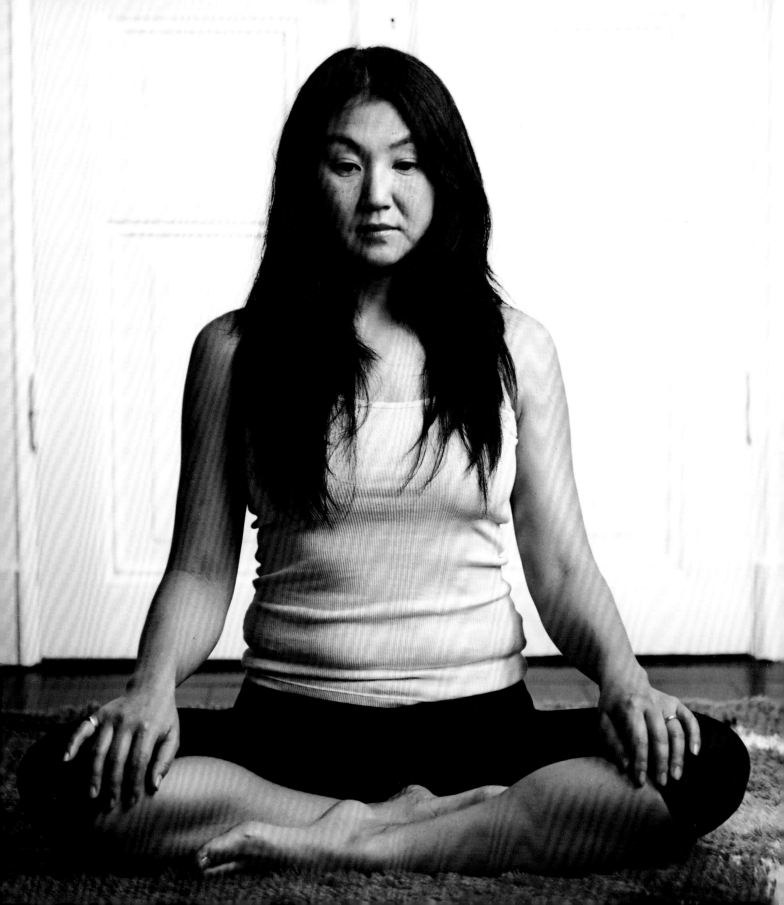

Pelvic Lift A

HOW TO DO IT
- Lie down on the floor on your back with your knees bent and your feet hip-distance apart on the ground. Rest your arms by your sides with the palms on the floor.
- Relax your shoulders and imagine that you are increasing the space between your ears and your shoulders. Lengthen your neck by tilting your chin to your chest.
- Press the feet into the floor, and engage the gluteus muscles on an exhale. Simultaneously engage the pelvic floor muscles. Repeat this a few times. If it feels good, move on to the next pelvic lift.

Pelvic Lift B

HOW TO DO IT
- Lift your hips and engage the pelvic floor muscles on an inhale; keep engaging as you breath out and stay lifted. Try to keep your inhales and exhales even. Take a few breaths like this.
- Slowly come down vertabra by vertabra on an exhale.
- Rest if this pose becomes too weight-bearing or uncomfortable. Lie still and breathe calmly and evenly.

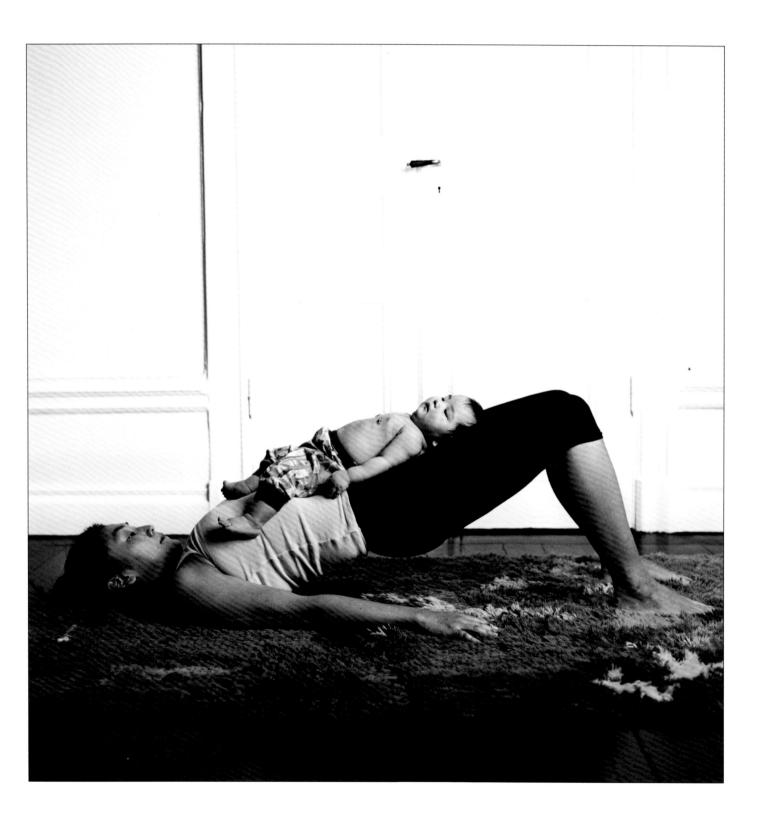

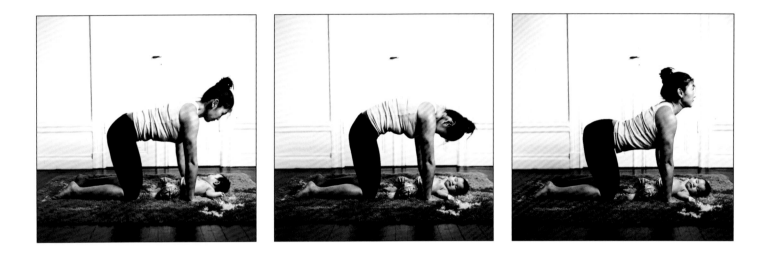

Pelvis Lift in Cat Pose

BENEFITS
This exercise strengthens the uterus and the pelvic floor muscles. This pose also relieves the pressure on the lumbar spine and strengthens your breath.

HOW TO DO IT
- Come onto all fours with your hands shoulder-width apart and your legs, knees, and feet hip-distance apart. Find the natural curve of the spine and make that your starting position.
- Exhale and round your back so that the small of the back is almost flat. You can almost feel how the uterus is pulled up when you simultaneously engage the pelvic floor muscles.
- Inhale and come back to the starting position and stay here for the exhale.
- On the next inhale, reach your chest up and lower your abdomen down. Lift the head and reach it back.
- Repeat these steps slowly several times. Rest in Adho Mukha Virasana/child's pose in between if you need to (see page 74).

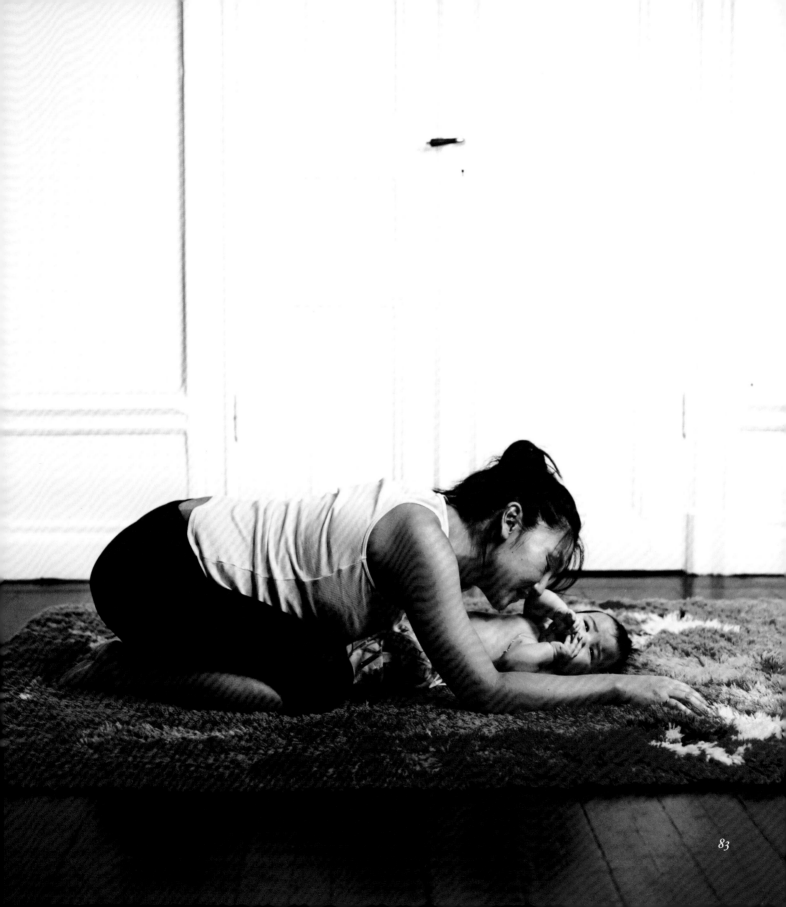

Chapter 8:
The Woman in Her 40s

You are in the middle of life. The years have passed. You have experienced sadness and joy. You have somehow understood that you are not immortal, and that you need to start taking great care of yourself. Everything matters all of a sudden, what you eat and how you eat it, if you work out or not. These are things that will make you or break you through the years. To invest in your health is the best retirement plan you can get and it is never too late to begin. Not only will you become stronger, more flexible, and more agile, but yoga will also affect your mind. You will cultivate patience, and yoga will prepare you to face life's changes with love, respect, and belief in yourself. It will strengthen you in all the choices you make, both good and the ones that aren't great. It is all right to not always succeed in everything you set out to achieve. You will learn to listen more to yourself, and not care so much about what everyone else thinks. You will learn to set boundaries and hopefully how to take one day at a time—stay present. Not tomorrow or yesterday. Now.

Yoga poses shown by author of the book

Karin Björkegren, 43 years

"To me yoga is the best retirement plan I could ever
get. I imagine myself as a happy and agile senior
citizen. Yoga has made me calmer, which helped
me to find a true joy that is grounded. Authentic."

85

The Woman in her 40s

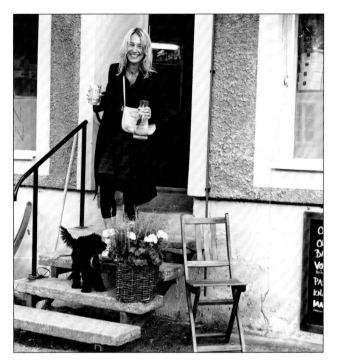

The Woman in the Middle of Life

Yes, that is exactly where I am and I have never felt more beautiful despite wrinkles, cellulite, and varicose veins. Not to mention gravity, which make most things sag, but I feel beautiful anyway. Perhaps because I am finally over forty years old and I have matured and realized that beauty is not about what you look like, but how you feel. I believe that it is thanks to my new love, my great friend, that I am able to get out of bed with confidence and observe my naked body in the mirror with kind eyes. Sure, I see the imperfections, but I no longer focus on them, instead I see myself as a whole. And life isn't really about appearance but about how you approach life in general. I have noticed a huge transformation in myself and others when it comes to this approach.

A Wandering Head

I have encountered plenty of women in the yoga community, both as a student and as a teacher. My very first teacher was in her forties when I began practicing ashtanga vinyasa yoga. She was so comfortable in her own body and it made her absolutely beautiful. I felt that I lacked that kind of confidence towards my own body.

I used to be like a huge head walking around aimlessly, not at all grounded. I only worked and stressed my way through life and had no clue that I needed to stop to take a breath and connect my mind and body.

Another teacher told me that she used to hate her belly before she started practicing yoga. It was a belly that had given birth to two children and that she considered so ugly that she would not even touch it to moisturize it with lotion. Today, she no longer apologizes for any of her imperfections. She wears tight pants and tops with confidence while instructing her students.

As a student, it is inspiring to see how these women that are over forty years old grab ahold of their lives and day after day roll out their yoga mats to confront themselves. I have heard stories about how yoga has transformed them into confident women that are not afraid to meet life's challenges. Yes, no wonder I almost sound religious when I speak about yoga. It does something to people. Yoga takes our values and thoughts and turns them upside down.

We Are Good Enough Just the Way We Are

As a teacher I witness what yoga does to women. Most of my students are women that are approaching their fifties. These are women with pretty low self-esteem, at least when it comes to their belief in their body's ability. Just like I was when I first started practicing. These women are stressed, with their shoulders tensed up all the way to their ears. Women that almost don't breathe, at least not deeply. But after just a few classes I see how these women start to settle into their own bodies. How their breath has deepened and how their inhales and exhales are even. All of a sudden they are using their entire lungs when they breathe.

I often have to remind my students that they are good enough just the way they are. It is perhaps a cliché, but it has to be repeated over and over so that it somehow manifests itself in the mind. Because it is the truth. We are good enough just the way we are. We don't need to be perfect—we just need to like who we are. But we sometimes need a little bit of help for that, because the pressure from the external world is powerful. Yoga is like a good friend that encourages you when your confidence runs short.

HONEY-INFUSED APPLE CIDER VINEGAR

Honey-infused apple cider vinegar in a glass of water can strengthen the body. Honey is calming and is said to be an aphrodisiac. Honey is full of nutrients and contains minerals, vitamins, and amino acids. According to ayurvedic principles it contains antibiotic properties but only in its raw, unheated state. Honey is also an excellent moisturizer and you can massage it into your skin for a refreshing face mask.

Utthita Trikonasana—Triangle Pose

BENEFITS
Many women have pains in their lower back once they are forty and over. Triangle pose stretches the spine along the sides as it activates the spinal nerves, which stimulates digestion. This pose stretches the entire side and strengthens the abdominal muscles.

HOW TO DO IT
- Inhale and on the exhale, step your right foot to the right and try to keep both legs straight and strong as you reach your right index and middle finger around your right big toe. If you can't reach the toes, grab hold of your ankle. Heels are in line with each other. Right foot is turned out 45 degrees.
- Try to create a straight line from your right foot up through the shoulders to the left hand. Stay like this for 5 breaths.
- Inhale and come up and turn the feet parallel to each other. Turn left foot out 45 degrees. Exhale and come down, grabbing your left big toe with left index finger and middle finger, or hold the ankle.
- Reach right arm up to the ceiling.
- Try to create a straight line between your left foot and up through the shoulders all the way up through your right hand. Take 5 long and calm breaths here.

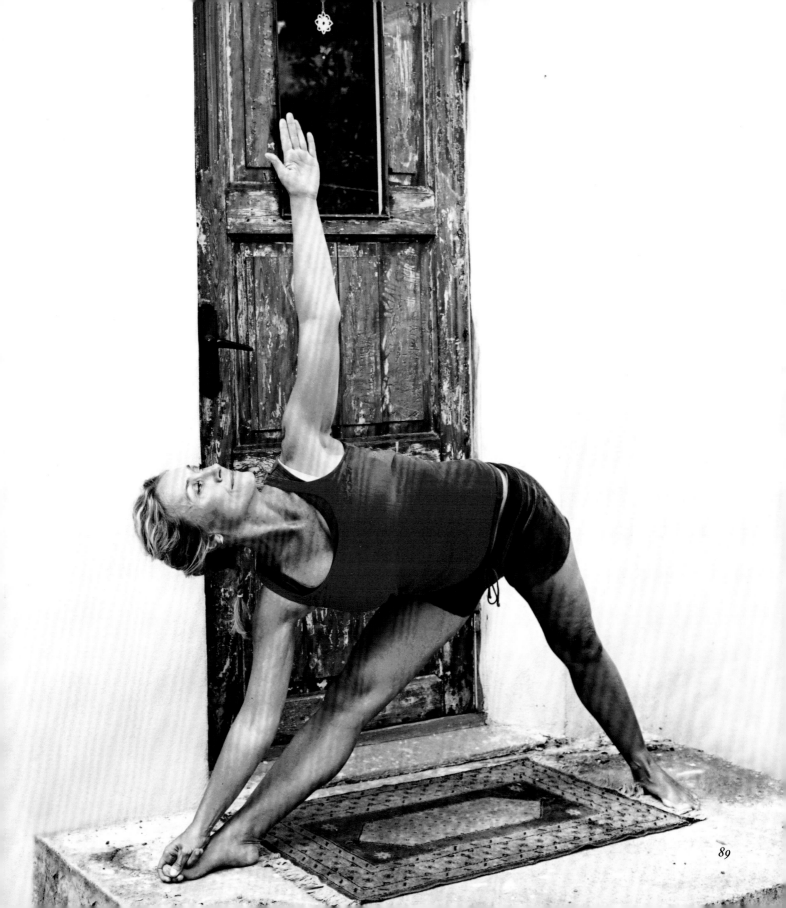

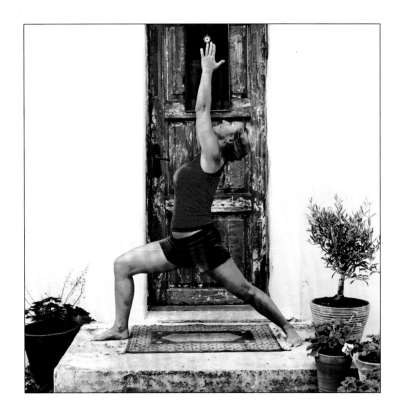

Virabhadrasana 1—Warrior Pose

BENEFITS
A versatile pose that strengthens the arms and legs. It is also tones the spine and diminishes tension in the shoulder blades and opens up the chest. It softens the pelvic region, improves digestion, and it can relieve pains related to menstruation.

HOW TO DO IT
• Stand with your legs wide apart and keep the feet parallel to each other. Turn out the right foot so that the foot and knee face in the same direction.
• Slightly turn in the left foot so that it is in line with the left hip and left knee. Your goal is to eventually keep your hips parallel.
• Bend the right knee into a 90 degree angle. Keep the back leg strong and straight by pressing down through the entire sole of the foot.
• Reach your arms up to the ceiling, but lower your shoulder and look towards your thumbs. Feel powerful like a warrior.
• Stay in this pose for 5–10 breaths. Switch legs and repeat on the other side.

Virabhadrasana 3—Airplane

BENEFITS
This pose charges you with energy and strengthens the legs, hips, and shoulders.

HOW TO DO IT
- Start out in warrior pose and bend your torso forward over the stretched right leg.
- Lift your left leg off the floor and straighten it behind you so that it is parallel to the floor.
- Lower the left hip so that it is in line with the right hip.
- Turn your left inner thigh in so that the toes point toward the ground, and stretch out through the left heel. Imagine a line of energy that extends all the way through the spine.
- Stay in this pose for 5–10 breaths and repeat on the other leg.

Dandasana—Staff Pose

BENEFITS

This pose strengthens the spine and the legs, and it prepares you for the next pose, Paschimottanasana.

HOW TO DO IT

• Exhale. Sit on the floor with legs straight out in front of you. Press the palms against the floor next to your hips.
• Lengthen your back, lift your chest up like you are opening up your heart, and tuck your chin slightly in towards your chest.
• Lift the heels off the floor.
• Sit like this for 5 deep breaths.

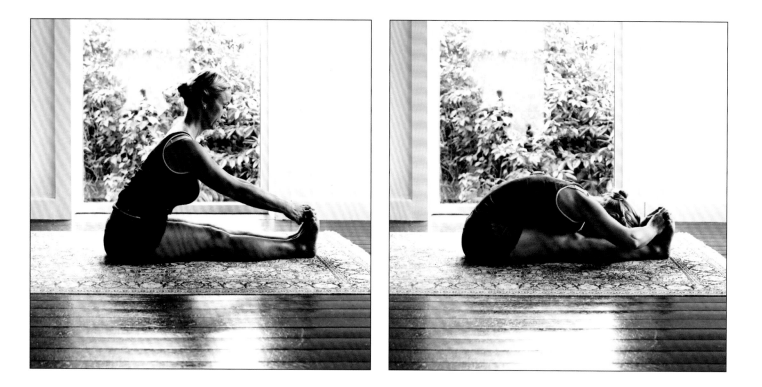

Paschimottanasana—Seated Forward Bend

BENEFITS

The seated forward bend lengthens the spine and creates space between the vertebrae, and hugs the internal organs in the abdominal area in addition to supplying them with oxygen and firing up the digestive organs.

HOW TO DO IT

• Exhale as you stretch your torso forward over the legs and grab the big toes with your thumb and index finger.
• Inhale and stretch up.
• Exhale, fold forward, and try to touch the knees with your chin. Don't try to reach the knees to the head because that will only make your back hunch too much. Instead, your goal is to reach your torso as far forward as possible, with knees and spine lengthening. Try to reach out and stretch forward from the tailbone. If you can't reach your toes, bend your knees slightly, or place your hands by your knees and carefully fold forward so that you feel that the bend is happening from the hip and not the spine.
• Stay like this for 5–10 deep breaths.

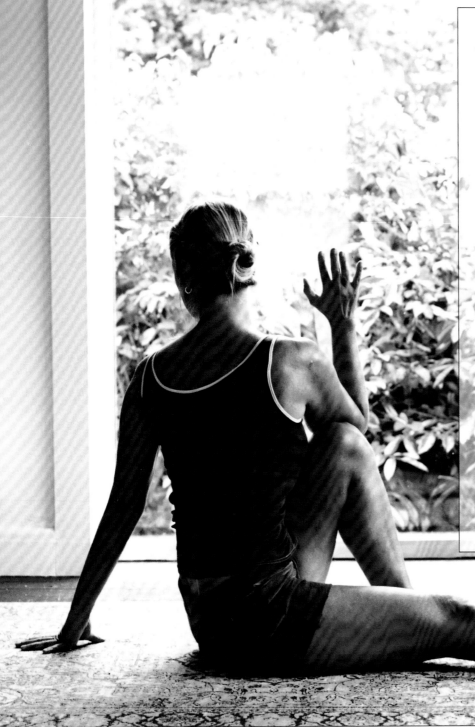

Marychasana C

BENEFITS

Spinal twists are movements that rotate the spine. Most other movements bend the spine back or forward, but the back doesn't get fully flexible until it bends sideways as well. The movement activates the nerves in the spine and the ligaments and is said to improve digestion. Keep the spine upright and maintain the shoulders level with each other in this twist. Keep the inhales and exhales even and twist a little bit deeper on each exhale.

HOW TO DO IT

- Sit on the floor.
- Inhale, bend the left leg and place the heel on the ground in line with left hip, while the right leg is extending forward on the floor with the foot flexed.
- Rotate the torso towards the bent left leg.
- Place the right elbow on the outside of the left knee so that you can feel your left side stretching out.
- Look over your left shoulder toward the back.
- Sit like this for 5 deep breaths. Switch the legs and repeat the twist on the other side.

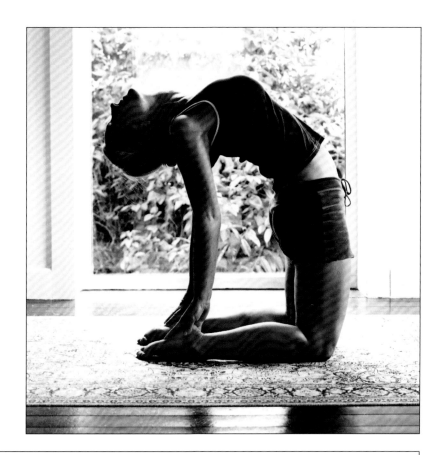

Ustrasana—Camel Pose

BENEFITS

Camel pose is great to strengthen the legs and stretch and open up the chest. It also tones the abdominal muscles. The opening of the chest contributes to the health of the lungs and the breath. It also improves blood circulation in the entire body.

HOW TO DO IT

- Stand on your knees.
- Inhale and lift the chest up.
- Exhale as you lean back and reach your arms behind you and grab the heels with your hands. It is paramount that you keep the legs engaged and strong. Make sure that the bend happens in the upper back as it is easy to bend in the lower back instead. Reach the head back and keep lifting and curling the chest open.
- If this pose is too intense for you, don't reach all the way back to your heels. Just lean as far back as is comfortable and breathe.

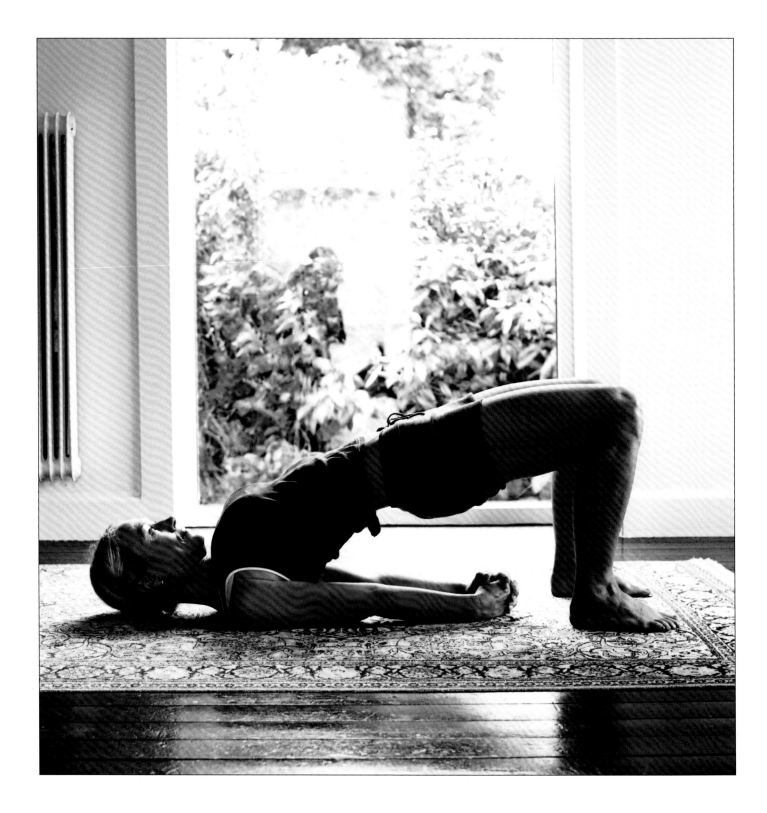

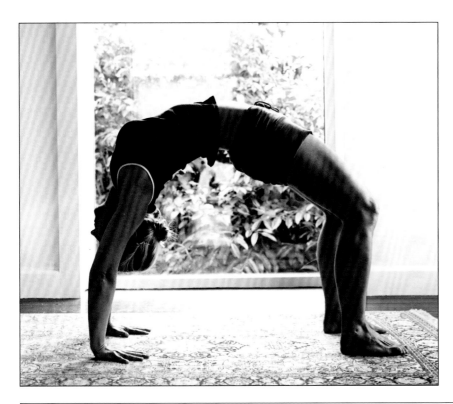

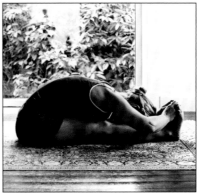

COUNTER POSE
- Sit up and stretch the legs out in front of you.
- Inhale and lengthen the spine and fold the torso over your legs on an exhale.
- Rest the heads on your knees. Breathe here for 5 long breaths. Allow your body to follow the breath.

Ardh Chakrasana—Half Wheel Pose

BENEFITS

This movement increases the flexibility in the spine. It opens up the shoulders and neck where one often accumulates tension, and it strengthens the abdomen. This pose is preparation for more advanced poses, such as full wheel pose/upward facing bow pose, and shoulder stand.

HOW TO DO IT
- Lie down on your back and bend the knees.
- Place the feet hip-distance apart so the toes are pointing straight in front of you.
- Place the arms along the sides of your body and lift the pelvis up. Press down through the feet and try to reach the pelvis to the ceiling.
- Clasp the hands behind your back and press the arms into the ground. Try to lift the chest up.
- Breathe in this pose for 5 breaths, come down, and rest for a few breaths. Repeat the pose 3 times.

ALTERNATIVE

Come into a full wheel pose from the half wheel pose, by placing your hands on each side of your head, fingers pointing towards your feet. Press down through the hands and feet, and lift up and come up to the top of your head. From there, lift all the way up stretching your arms and legs straight as you lift the pelvis higher.

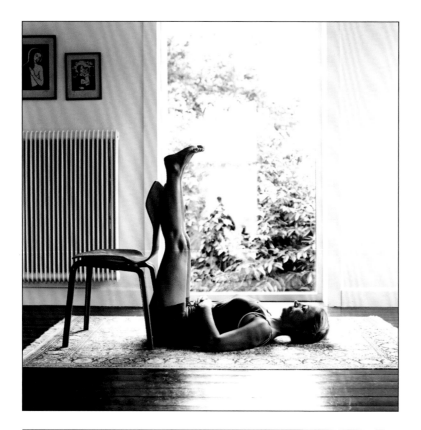

Sarvangasana—Shoulderstand—The Queen of Yoga Poses

BENEFITS
This pose is worth practicing every day as it is calming and regulates the hormones.

HOW TO DO IT
- To keep the neck relaxed and in its natural curve, please fold a blanket and place under the shoulders so that the neck is lifted away from the floor. Lie on your back. Bend the knees.
- Lift your butt, legs and hips up into the air. Support your back with your hands. The legs might lean a bit over your head in the beginning. Eventually, with regular practice, you will be able to keep the legs right above the shoulder blades. Keep the legs together. Don't turn the neck, once in shoulder stand the neck should remain still.
- Stay in this pose for up to 25 breaths.
- When you come out of the pose, slowly roll your spine down to the floor, vertebra by vertebra.

ALTERNATIVE
If your neck or shoulders are hurting or if you are menstruating, do this pose against a chair.

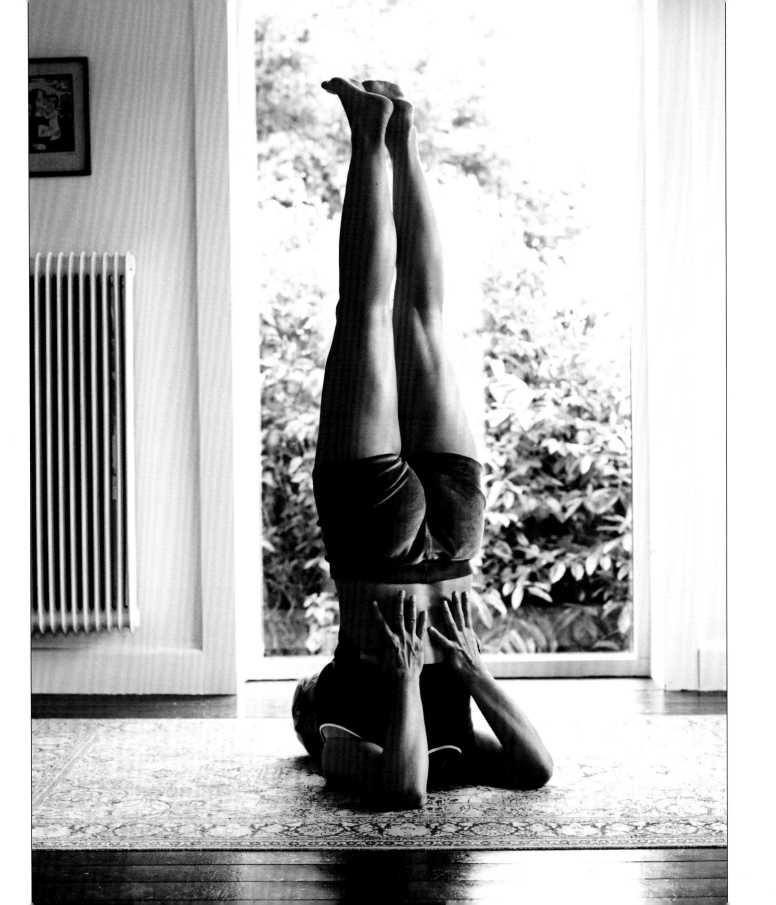

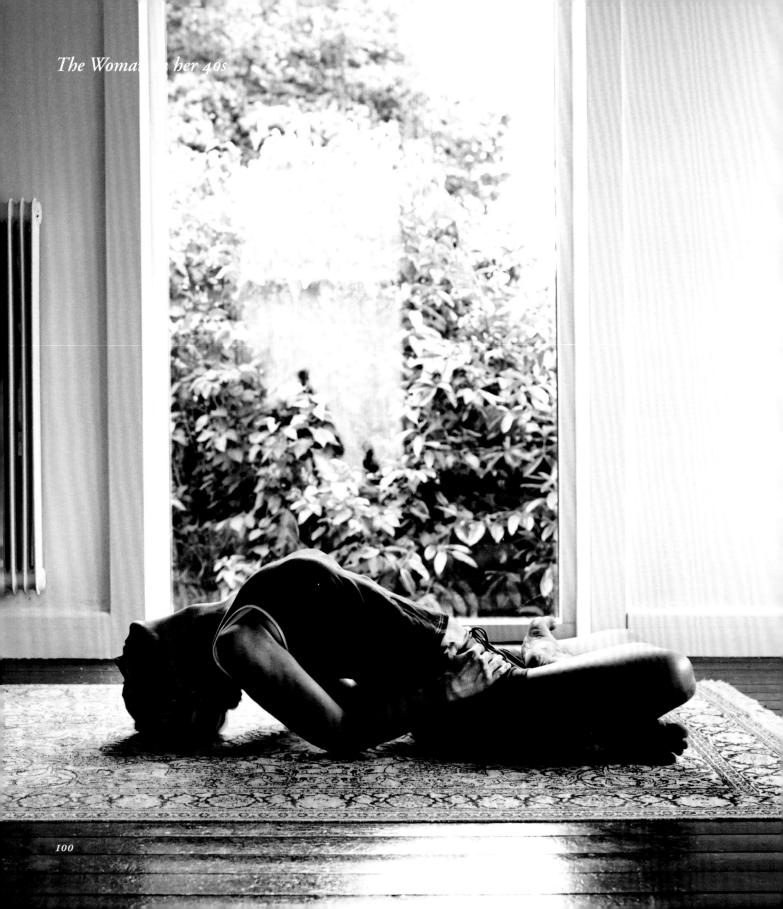

Matsyasana—Fish Pose with Crossed Legs

BENEFITS

It is good to do the fish pose after any of the shoulder stands. You can either do the kinder fish pose (see page 59), or you could take a fish pose in a cross-legged position. This pose opens up the chest and improves breathing as the lungs are stretched.

HOW TO DO IT

• Lie down on your back with your legs in a cross-legged position. Lift your chest up by supporting yourself onto your elbows. Imagine that you are opening up your heart to the sky. Expose the throat up as you tilt the back of the head back and down into the floor. Think of lengthening the spine backwards into a bow shape.

• To make this pose more challenging, you can lift your elbows off the floor and place them on your knees. Be aware of where you keep your shoulders. Try to lengthen the space between your shoulders and your ears.

• You can stay like this for 5–10 deep breaths. Come out of it immediately if you feel any discomfort in the neck. Other wise, come out of the pose mindfully with your neck and shoulders against the floor, and hug your knees into your chest to stretch out the back again. Get in and out of the pose slowly, and use the breath to guide you in the movements.

Chapter 9: Menopause

Yoga can reduce the hormonal imbalances that occur during menopause. Yoga soothes the issues that are often experienced by women during this transitional period.

IT IS SAID THAT WOMEN ENTER THEIR TRANSITIONAL AGE, or menopause, when they are between forty-five and fifty-five years old. It usually starts a year or two before a woman's last menstruation, and continues for about 5 years. During this time of transition, the hormonal balance changes vastly in the body. The ovaries no longer produce as much of the female hormones estrogen and progesterone. The reduced amount of estrogen contributes to issues such as sweats, hot flashes, trouble sleeping, and mood swings.

Yoga does not only affect bones and muscles, but also organs and glands. That is why yoga is such an excellent form of exercise during menopause to help calm your body and mind. Yoga poses balance the body and mind and positively affect your health.

Yoga helps women to deal with menopause mentally, but it is also inspiring spiritually. Menopause is a natural and very important experience in a woman's life. Just as important as your very first menstruation and the prospect of becoming a mother. Just like the menstruation is a bridge between being a girl and becoming a woman, menopause is the road that leads to the wise woman's world.

The Wise Woman's World

Amongst the Indians, a woman could only become a shaman or a medicine woman once she had passed menopause. This transitional period is an opportunity for a woman to bloom fully into the position of the powerful, creative, and wise woman that she in fact is.

It is the time to really feel and think about what is important in your life. Listen to your inner voice and allow yourself to slow down. Enjoy your newly found opportunity to look inside of you and to stay present. Yoga can help you to pause so that you take the time to enjoy yourself and your body.

Many of the poses in the chapter about menstruation are also effective to soothe the issues experienced during menopause.

Yoga poses shown by yoga teacher

Britta Larsson-Jones, 51 years old

"My first encounter with yoga was eleven years ago when a friend of a friend, my yoga teacher, Maria, returned from India and began to teach. We were a little group of perhaps five students, and since then yoga has expanded. I fell in love with yoga and today it is part of my life. It has taught me to listen to my body and to hear what makes it feel good. Yoga is meditative and creates inner peace and presence. It has also made me more flexible and balanced. Yes, yoga simply makes me a happier woman."

Menopause

Menopause comes from the Greek term mensis, which means month and is defined as the time of the last menstruation. The time before and after menopause, the woman is in her climacteric. The time for menopause varies but on average it occurs when a woman is fifty-one years old. At least 95 percent of women have passed their menopause by the age of fifty-five, and at fifty-eight very few of them still menstruate. When the last menstruation is approaching, the amount of estrogen is slowly reduced in the blood, and about five years after the last period, the estrogen levels are constantly low, just like before puberty. Menopause happens when there are no more egg cells in the ovaries. That is why the ovaries lose their ability to react to the hormones that stimulate the ova to become fertile eggs.

Health Tip: OATMEAL

Eat a bowl of oatmeal a day and sprinkle generously with cinnamon. The spice is a great circulation booster and is especially effective during menopause. Cinnamon is also said to increase appetite—both sexually and gastronomically. Oats lower cholesterol in the blood, and contain anti-depressive components and relieve fatigue.

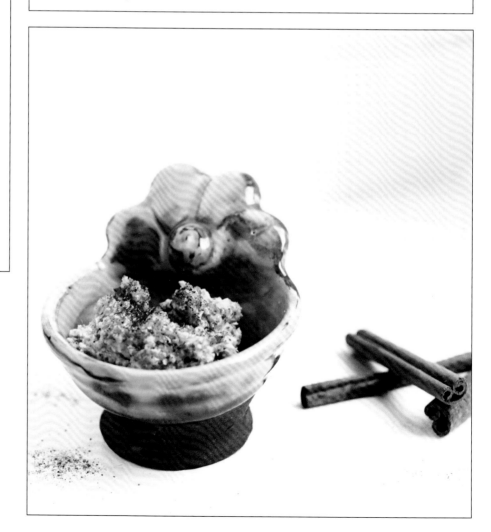

A study conducted by the International Journal of Neuroscience found that a group of fifty-year-olds that had practiced transcendental meditation for over five years had a biological age twelve years lower than the control groups.

Adho Mukha Svanasana—Downward Facing Dog

BENEFITS

This pose stretches the entire backsides of the legs and the gluteus muscles. It lengthens the spine, and it softens the areas around the shoulder blades, the shoulders, and the arms. The blood flows to the brain and the pose also strengthens the heart by calming the heartbeats. Downward facing dog pose is said to increase self-esteem, and to carefully stimulate the nervous system, calm the mind, and be a good pose for women going through menopause. It is also said to stabilize the blood pressure and counteract harde-ning of the arteries. This powerful asana influences all the systems in the body, and is cooling while energy enhancing. It counteracts brittleness in the bones in the hands, wrists, arms, and shoulders, and it prevents night sweats and hot flashes.

HOW TO DO IT

- Sit down onto your knees, fold your torso forward towards the floor, and reach your arms straight out in front of you on the floor.
- Tuck your toes under and come into downward facing dog. Now you have the correct distance between your feet and your hands. Keep the hands shoulder-width apart and the feet hip-distance apart.
- Lift the butt towards the ceiling, but don't arch your back. Dist-ribute weight evenly over your hands and feet. Strive to reach the heels to the ground.
- Gaze in between your feet. Stay here for 5–10 breaths.

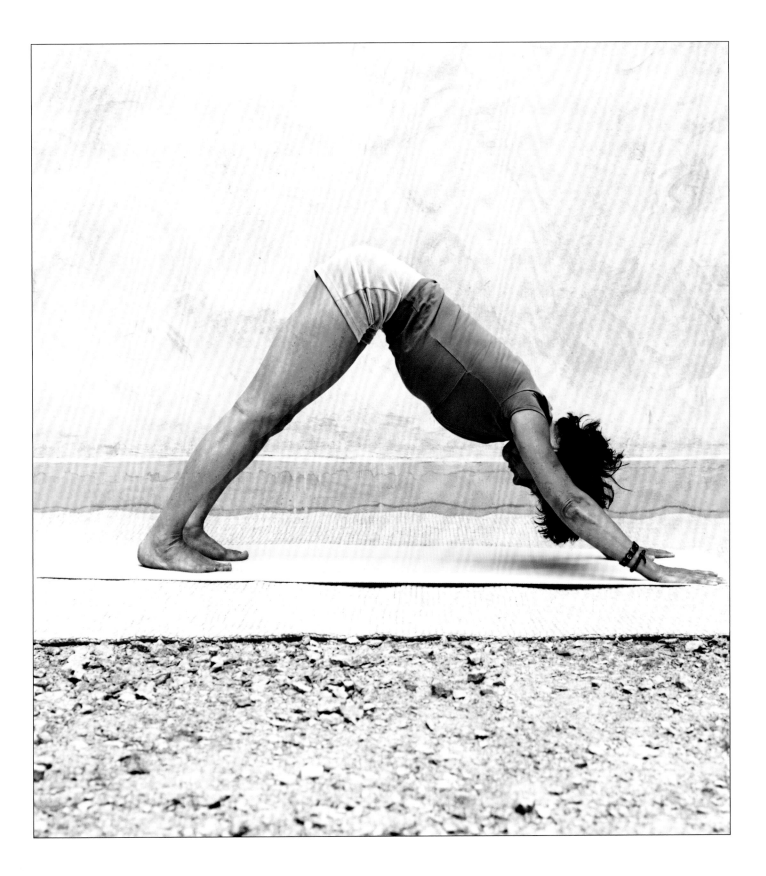

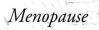

Ardha Chandrasana—Half Moon

BENEFITS
This pose rotates the spine, which strengthens the entire spine and increases flexibility. It can correct imbalances in the shoulders and reduce sciatica issues. The circulation in the feet is boosted and digestion improves, and it can help to relieve issues such as heartburn and a gassy stomach. The uterus is stimulated and the blood circulation in the stomach improves.

HOW TO DO IT
• Begin by standing with your back against a wall. Place a block by the wall for support.
• Turn your right foot so that it is parallel to the wall.
• Place your right hand on the block and reach your right hand up so that it extends away from the shoulder directly over the right arm. Imagine that you lengthen your spine so that you don't drop your chin.
• Turn your neck and look towards your left hand.
• Lift your left leg so that it is parallel to the ground.
• Hold this pose for 20 seconds, and repeat on the other side.

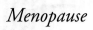

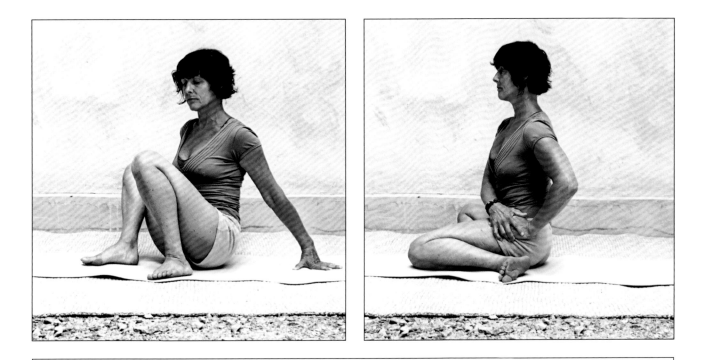

Hip Openers

BENEFITS
This pose may look simple, but it is very effective. It stretches out the hips and the groin and increases blood circulation to the hip and pelvic region.

HOW TO DO IT
- Sit down and bend both knees and angle your left leg to the side. Keep the left foot as close to the left thigh as possible.
- Bend right leg back and angle the right foot away from your left hip, and bring both knees down to the right. Sit like this for a moment. Your goal should be to reach the entire buttocks to the ground. This pose attends to any tightness in the hips.
- Bring both knees up, but keep the feet on the ground and roll knees down to the other side to repeat the pose.
- If you feel tightness in the muscles, imagine that you guide your breath to it to undo tensions.
- Stay for 10–15 breaths on each side.

Bhujangasana—Cobra

BENEFITS

This pose may look simple but it takes a lot of determination and strength to perform it. Every time you inhale, the organs in your abdomen benefit from the massage that occurs when the belly expands against the floor. Both the spine and the nervous system are activated positively. This pose counteracts stress and increases energy. It opens up the chest and increases body temperature. This asana strengthens the pelvic floor muscles and gives you power. In yoga, the goal is to make the spine flexible when bending forward, back, and to the sides. According to an old Chinese saying, a flexible spine is the key to a long life. This pose strengthens and stabilizes the spine and increases the circulation in the back muscles.

HOW TO DO IT

• Lie down on your stomach, your forehead resting on the floor. Place the feet hip-distance apart. Press down through the big toe and the little toe, heels pointing towards the ceiling. Press the tops of the feet into the ground.
• Place the hands a bit in front of your chest (eventually the hands should be directly underneath the shoulders on the lift) and lift the chest forward and up. In the beginning, before the back is so flexible, keep the hands more in front of the chest so you do not over-stretch the back.
• Do not draw the shoulders up, but try to soften them by increasing the space between the ears and the shoulders.
• Take 5–8 breaths and come down to rest. Try to stay present and resilient in this pose, and lengthen evenly through the spine, all the way up through the neck.
• Repeat 2–3 times.

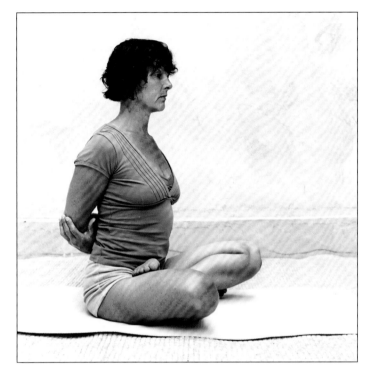 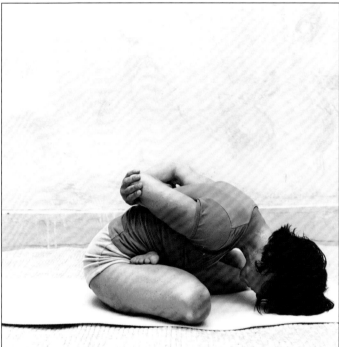

Yoga Mudra—Sitting Forward Bend

BENEFITS

Yoga mudra quiets the mind and is a preparatory pose for meditation. It has a calming and harmonic affect on the body. It stimulates the back and the intestines, and it helps to relieve constipation.

HOW TO DO IT

• Sit in a cross-legged position. If it is too uncomfortable you can sit on a bit of height, and that usually relieves the back. Try to find the highest point on your sit bones and imagine that you lengthen the spine up to the ceiling.

• Lengthen the spine all the way through the neck and slightly tuck the chin to your chest without dropping the neck. Feel how your chest lifts and expands and how your shoulders relax.

• Grab your elbows behind your back. Sit like this for 10 breaths, then fold your torso forward over your legs and rest your chin or forehead against the floor.

• Come up to sitting again.

Upavistha Konasana

BENEFITS

This pose stretches out the backside of the thighs and the hips and it also strengthens and straightens the spine. It improves circulation in the hips, strengthens the pelvic floor muscles, and is said to stimulate the intestines. The circulation in the pelvic region improves, which stimulates the uterus.

HOW TO DO IT

- Sit on the floor with your legs wide apart. Place your hands in front of you or on the legs and walk your fingertips forward so that you can lay your chest on the ground if that is possible. Make sure that you bend at the hip and not at the back.
- Lie like this and breathe for 3–4 minutes.

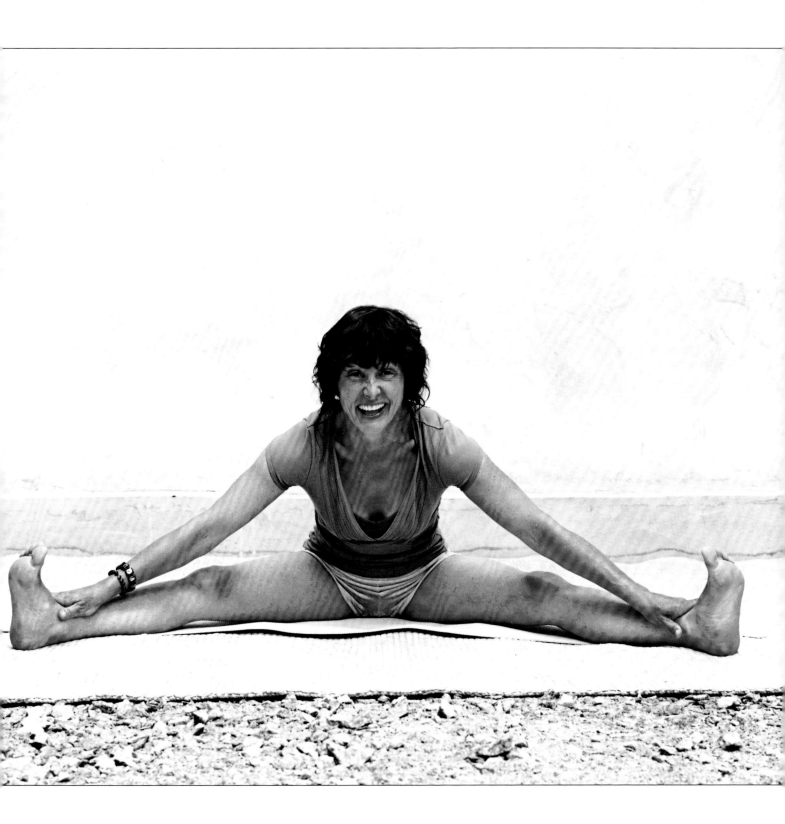

Sithali—Cooling Breath

BENEFITS
This is a cooling breathing technique that has a calming effect, and it is said to purify the blood and be good to counteract high blood pressure. So when the hot flashes come over you—or hot summer days—you can use sithali breathing to cool down.

HOW TO DO IT
• Stick the tongue out slightly and curl up the sides of the tongue so it is shaped into a pipe, and inhale through it while making a quiet hissing sound.
• Hold your breath for a moment before you exhale through the nose.

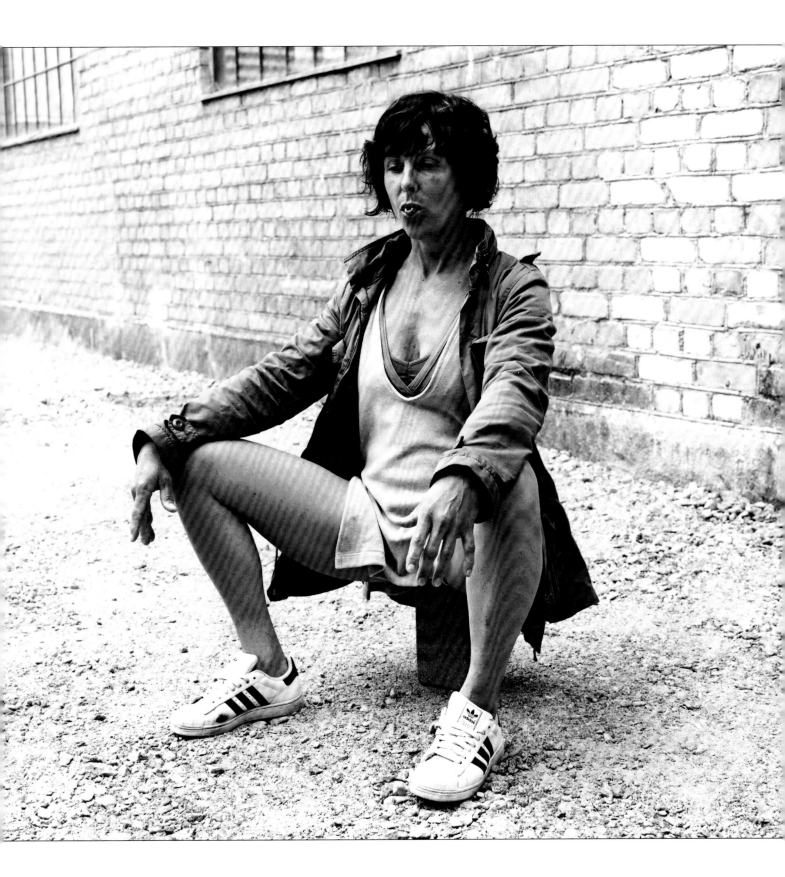

Chapter 10: The Woman in Her 50s–60s-plus

You are never too old for yoga. In fact, the older you get, the more you will benefit from yoga. It is possible that a younger practitioner has a stronger body, but she does not posses the same wisdom, the psychological and philosophical side that is so much more developed in the older yoga practitioner. You probably bring a certain amount of patience into your yoga practice—and allow it the time that it requires.

Yoga is your attitude towards yourself, your body, and to life in general. You will notice a big difference just after a few times that you practice yoga. It is NEVER too late to start. You can let the aging process become the best stage of your life by devoting time to your mind and body, which yoga really helps you to do. Many of the issues that one can experience with aging, such as poor blood circulation, problems with balance, digestion, or sleep, are often caused by the fact that we do not move enough, eat unhealthy, or only use shallow breathing.

I have said it before, but good things need to be repeated. Yoga is your very best retirement plan, as being physically active is important throughout life. Many older people consider yoga to be unusually strengthening, even after a few classes. You will notice that you sleep better, that your digestion improves, and that you gain more energy and become more focused. Yoga can be adjusted to your physical level, and advance as you gain more strength and flexibility. Yoga's greatest strength is that it will make you feel relaxed as you become more energized.

The yoga poses are shown by yoga teacher

Zoila Ravanti, 55 years old

"When I was seventeen years old, I found
a yoga book in my aunt's bookshelf. It
awakened my curiosity. Yoga keeps me
healthy and strong. It brings me mental
stability, joy, inspiration, calm, and peace.
Yoga also helps me to connect with the
deeper nuances of myself."

119

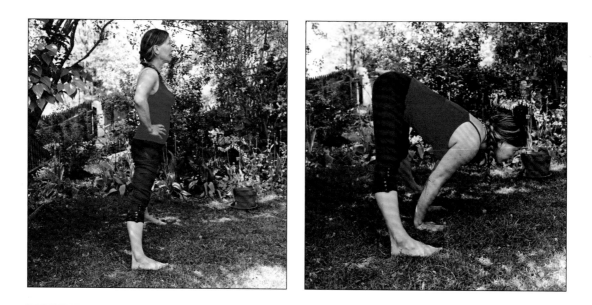

Prasarita Padottanasana A—Wide-legged Forward Bend

BENEFITS
This pose is said to increase joy and self-esteem. It strengthens the legs, reduces high blood pressure, and is good for stress related headaches.

HOW TO DO IT
- Step your right leg out to the right. The feet should be about 3 feet apart and parallel. We often have a tendency to walk and stand with our feet turned out, so make sure that the heel turns out a bit instead so that the outside of the foot is straight.
- Inhale, reach your back/chest, exhale and fold torso forward. Place the hands shoulder-width apart on the same line as the feet—if this is feasible for you.
- Lengthen the back and try to reach your head to the floor. Separate the shoulders from the head and reach your sit bones towards the ceiling. This forward bend stretches the backside of the thighs and is a preparatory pose for headstand.
- Stay in this pose for 5–10 calm and deep breaths.
- Keep the hands on the floor, inhale and lengthen your back all the way to your neck.
- Exhale.
- On an inhale, place the hands on your waist and come up with a straight back.

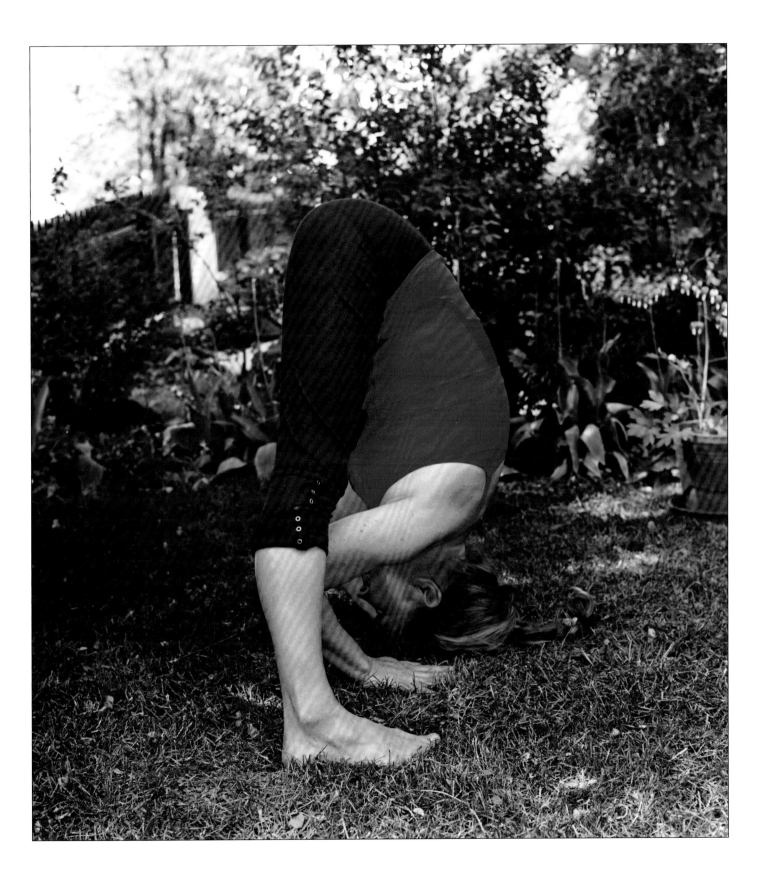

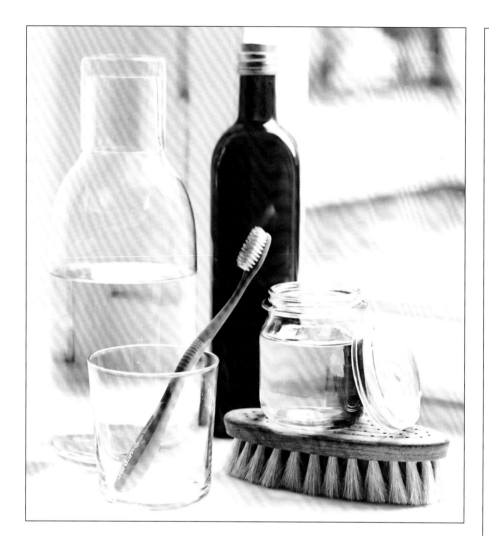

Health Tip

According to ayurveda, the Indian medical system, cleansing the tongue with a tongue scraper is an important ritual for health. You can even use your toothbrush to cleanse the tongue. During the night we collect bacteria in the mouth and the throat. Instead of swallowing the germs when you eat or drink in the morning, it is better to cleanse the tongue and brush the teeth first.

Wait 15 minutes after your yoga practice before you drink a glass of room temperature water. You can put out a pitcher of water the night before so that it is the perfect temperature in the morning.

Dry brush the entire body to jumpstart the blood circulation in the body. You can use an old-fashioned soft scrubbing-brush.

Moisturize your body with almond oil before you take a shower. It easily penetrates the skin and is rich in vitamin E, which is yummy for the skin.

Take care of your feet—your foundation. Moisturize them with olive oil. Cover with plastic bags and socks, and leave for a moment to let the olive oil soften the feet.

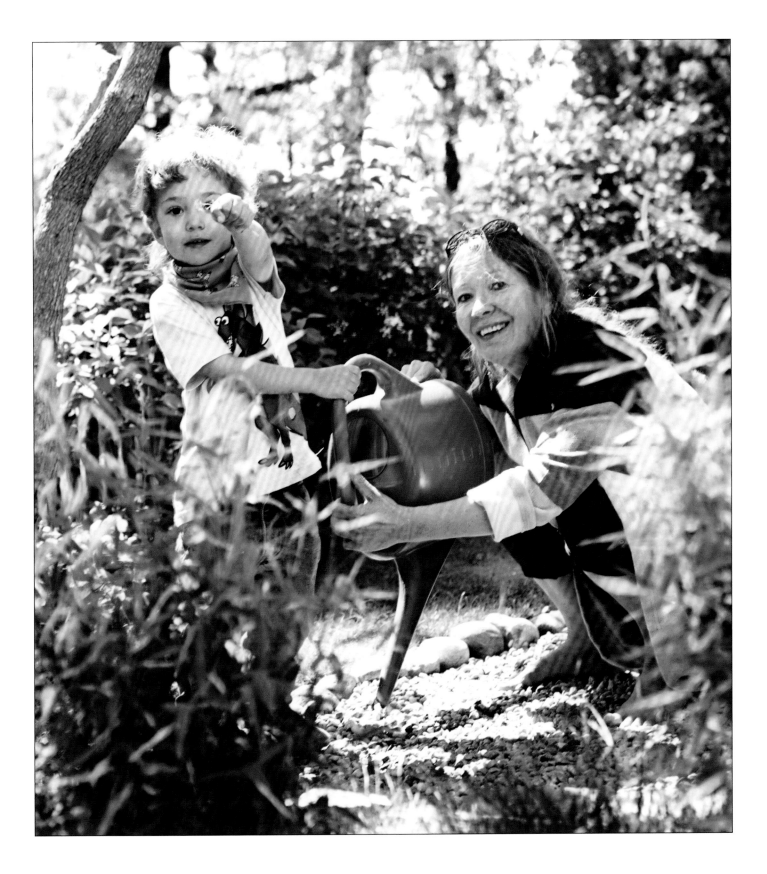

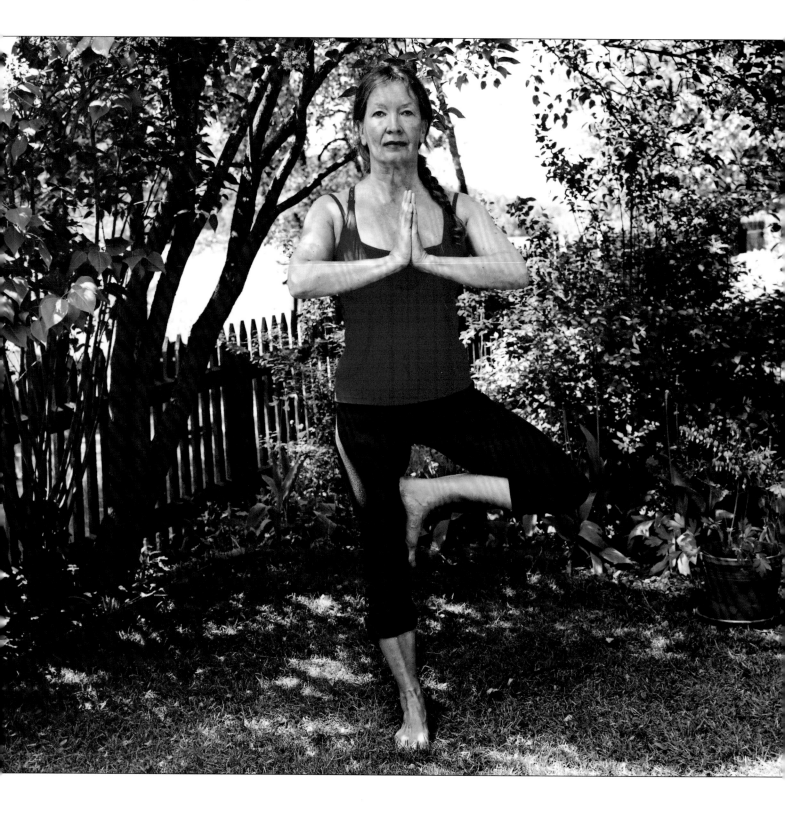

Vrikshasana—Tree Pose

BENEFITS

This pose is good for balance, which decreases a little bit with each year that passes. Good equilibrium counteracts accidental falls, which are common among older people. This asana improves your concentration so that you become more focused. It also strengthens your knees and ankles.

HOW TO DO IT

- Mountain pose (see page 66) is the foundation for all standing poses, where you stand firmly on the ground—like a mountain. Begin by standing with both feet parallel and hip-distance apart. Find your midline, pay attention to how you are standing. Are you perhaps leaning more on one foot? Hanging more to one hip? Imagine that you have three points underneath your feet. You press down through the big toes, the little toes, and the heels as you lift the arches of the feet.
- Try to keep the midline straight, even as you lift your left knee.
- Place the left foot on the right inner thigh. The big toe should point towards the ground and the goal is to keep the bent knee in line with the hips.
- In the beginning you can reach your arms out to the sides to keep your balance. When you feel more balanced you can bring the palms together in front of your chest, like in namaste, a salute.
- If it feels good, you can advance the pose by reaching your arms over your head, but keep the shoulders soft and relaxed.
- You can stay in this pose for 10–15 breaths. Switch legs and repeat on the other side.

Utthita Parshvakonasana —Extended Side Angle Pose

BENEFITS
Strengthens the legs, the knees, and the shoulder region. This pose is said to counteract back pains and makes your hips more flexible.

HOW TO DO IT
- Stand with your feet wide apart and parallel. Turn your right foot out and bend the right knee into a 90 degrees angle. If the knee bends past the toes, make your feet step wider apart so that the knee is directly over your ankle.
- Press down through your left foot, through the entire sole of the foot, so the left leg is engaged and strong.
- Place your right elbow on your left knee. Open up the chest, feel a little lift—imagine that you are opening up the heart to the sky —and take your left arm around your back to grab the inside of the right thigh.
- Look over your left shoulder, stretch the spine all the way to your neck.
- Stay in this pose for 5–10 breaths, and repeat on the other side.

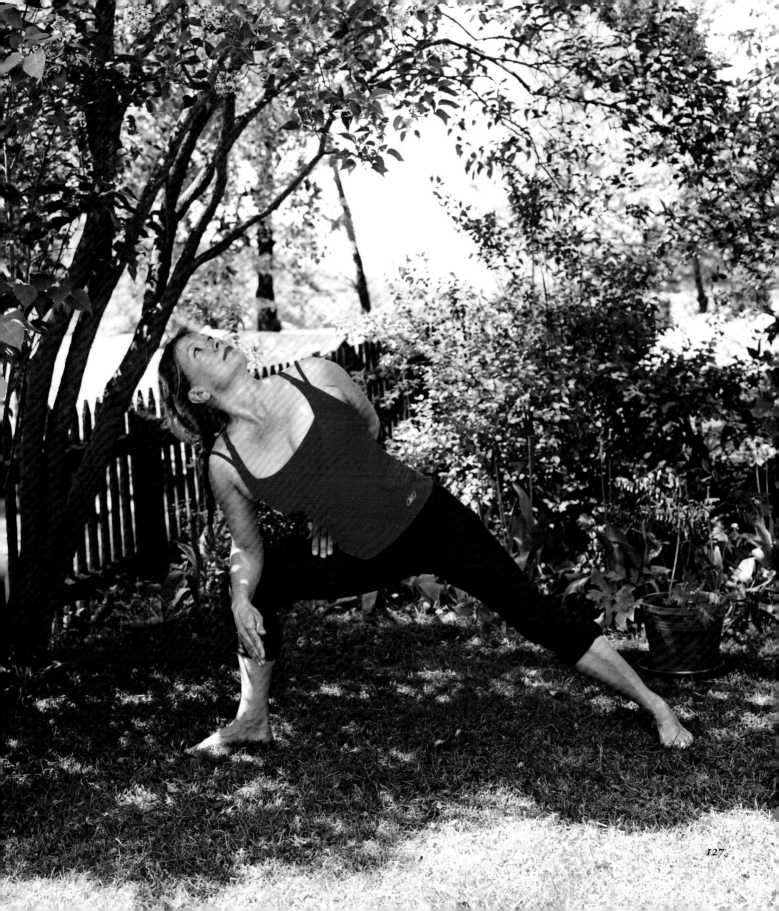

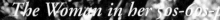

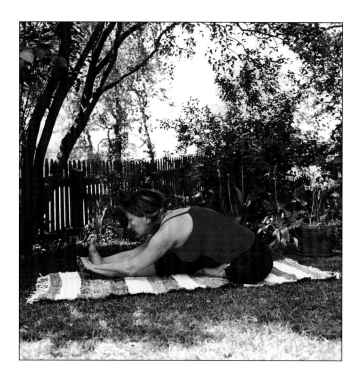

Janu Shirshasana A

BENEFITS
This pose straightens out the lumbar spine and opens up the hips, which is good for the entire pelvic region.

HOW TO DO IT
• Sit on the floor and straighten the right leg in front of you. Activate the leg by flexing the foot.
• Bend the left leg and let the left foot come to the inside of the left thigh, touching it if possible.
• Stretch out through your spine and lift the breast bone. Exhale and fold your torso over your right leg. Try to keep the buttocks on the floor.

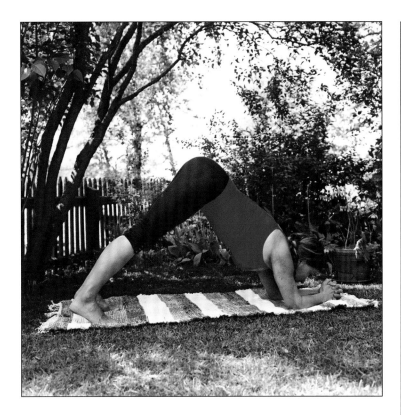

Plank Pose

BENEFITS
Builds up and strengthens the shoulders, neck, abdomen, back, and legs. In this pose you engage all the muscles that you need when getting into a headstand, so it is a good pose to prepare the body to stand on the head, but also to counteract tired shoulders and bad posture.

BENEFITS
- Stand on your knees. Place the elbows on the ground and reach the forearms in front of you. Clasp the hands and come into a downward facing dog on your forearms.
- Engage the navel in and activate the legs and the abdomen so that you have control over your body.
- On the exhale: shift your body forward and lower your body like a plank, without dropping the pelvis, and don't lower all the way to the ground.
- On the inhale: press down through the elbows and lift your hips into downward facing dog again.
- Repeat as many times as you can handle, but think about engaging the navel the entire time.
- Rest if you notice that your back is hanging to the ground so that you are over-arching the lumbar spine.

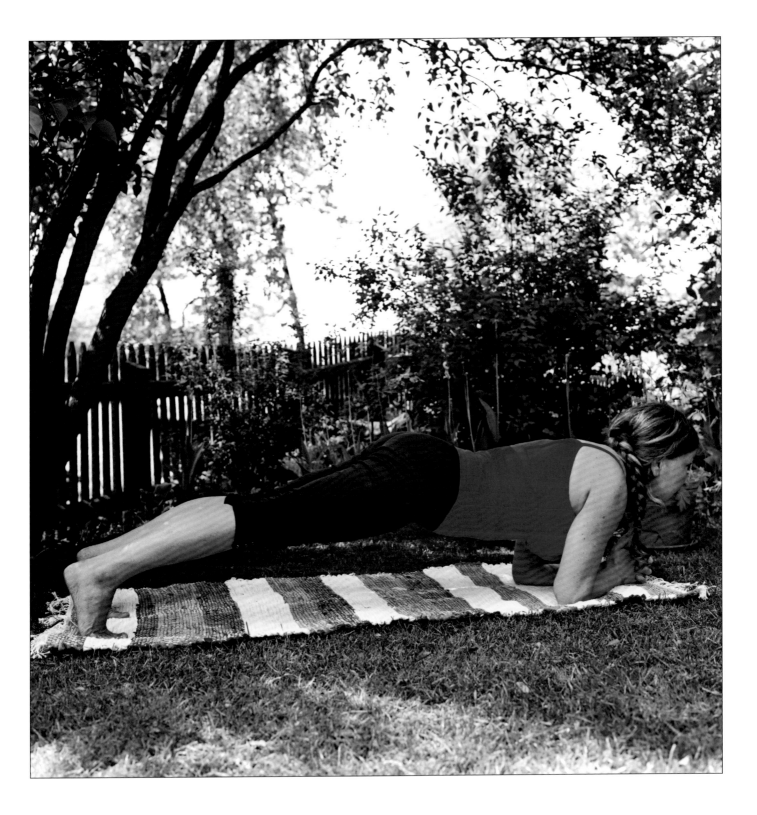

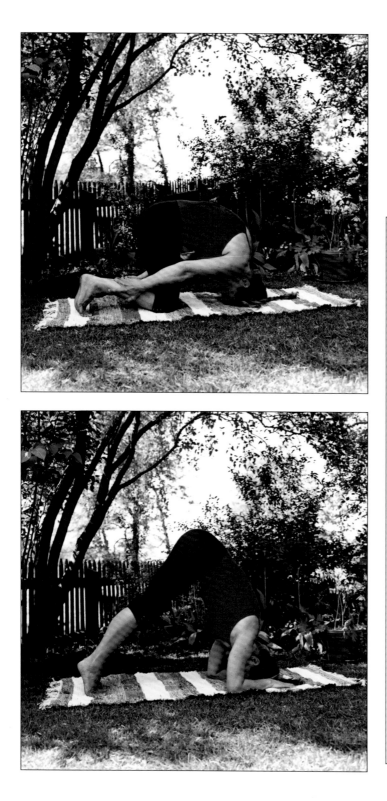

Hashankasana—Hare Pose

BENEFITS

Headstand is called the king of yoga poses, but it is also a very powerful and difficult asana. Before your body is ready for headstand, you will benefit from practicing hare pose and plank pose (see page 130), to build up strength and balance for headstand. When you stand on the head, more blood flows to the brain than in any other pose. It provides cells and tissues with nutrients and oxygen. Your focus increases, which can be helpful during studies, or mental work. The headstand is a preparatory pose for meditation. The entire body benefits from the stimulated circulation and the increased oxygen in the blood and relieves the heart from pressure.

HOW TO DO IT

- Start in child's pose (see page 74).
- Sit on your knees.
- Fold the torso forward.
- Lift the butt up high, inhale and roll onto the crown of the head. You can hold your feet with your hands.
- Stay here for 25 breaths. When it is time for headstand, let an experienced yoga teacher guide you into the pose.

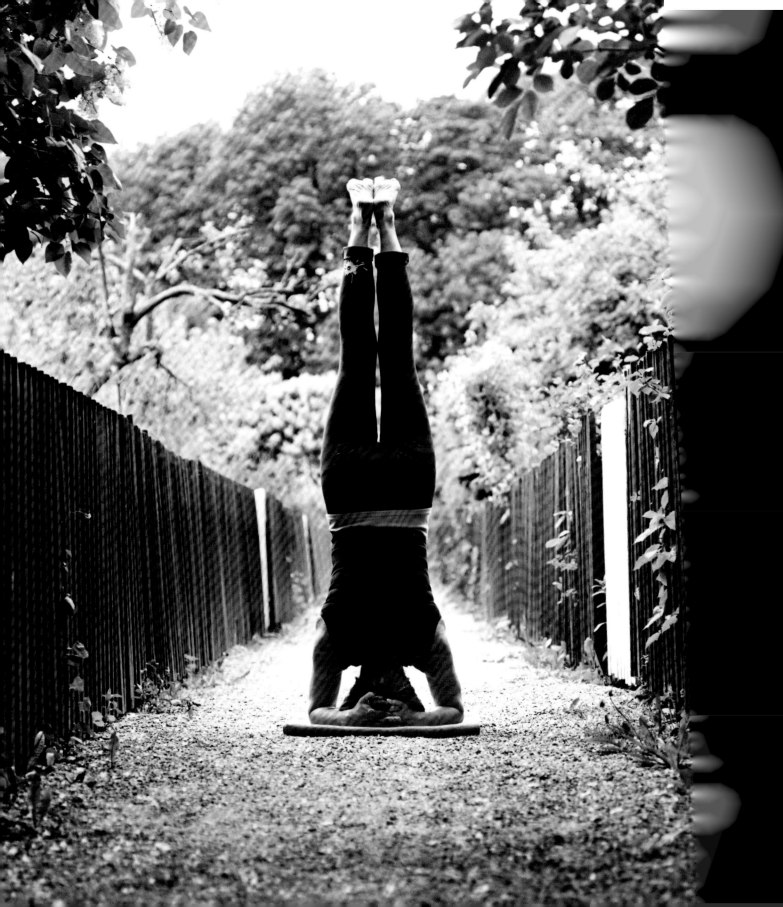

Chapter 11: Fit Yoga into Your Daily Routine

In the beginning I couldn't fathom how it was possible to fit a one to two hour- long yoga routine into the day, especially every day. I started out slowly, with one class a week. It soon increased to twice a week, and then I started to go to classes on some weekends. When life felt hectic because of issues at work or trouble in personal relationships, yoga became like a good friend to lean on. It was so nice to go to a class, roll out my mat, and stop thinking about all the things spinning in my head. That is when I decided to delve into yoga whole-heartedly—I began assisting several teachers and after a while I was teaching too. Yoga made me change my lifestyle pretty radically. But that doesn't have to be the case for everyone.

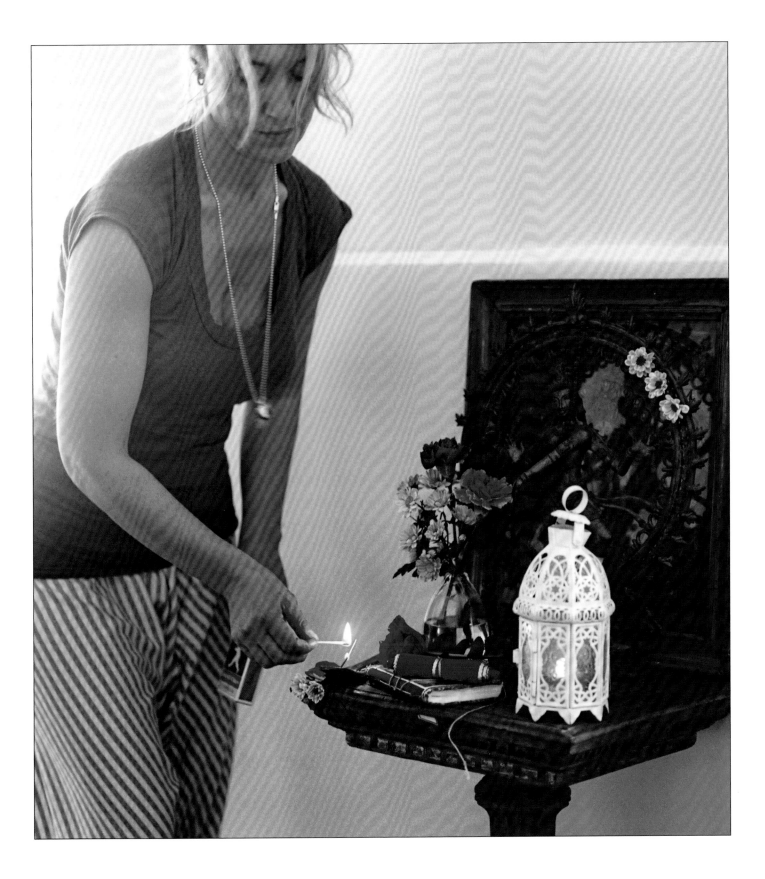

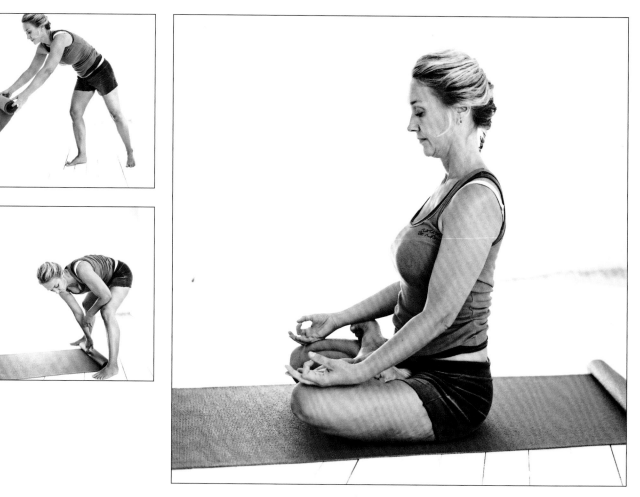

How often should I practice yoga?

Take it slow and let yoga take up as much room as possible. I usually answer that once a week is better then nothing, but if you practice even just a few sun salutations during the rest of the week, you will notice a bigger transformation. Never let yoga become a stressful moment in your life. That defeats the purpose of practicing. Yoga is there to enlighten your life, not to take over your life. It can easily become that way when you first start practicing. You become euphoric over what yoga can accomplish. It becomes like a discovery journey. You fall in love with yoga. That was at least my experience. My friends probably viewed me as a bore when I started going to bed at 10 p.m. on a Saturday night,

just so that I could get up early on Sunday morning to practice yoga. At first I found it unfortunate that none of my closest friends wanted to practice yoga, or that they didn't take it as seriously as I do. Today, eight years later, I am grateful that they stood by my side and listened to all my yoga talk. After a while that initial obsession disappears and yoga is just something that you do, just like you brush your teeth in the morning. It has become a habit to me. You can live life with yoga in it, but yoga is not life. Life continues to happen when you step off your yoga mat. Even if you practice six days a week, how you approach life, yourself, and others when you leave the yoga class is just as important as practice. Continue to live your life like you have, but add your new habit into it—yoga.

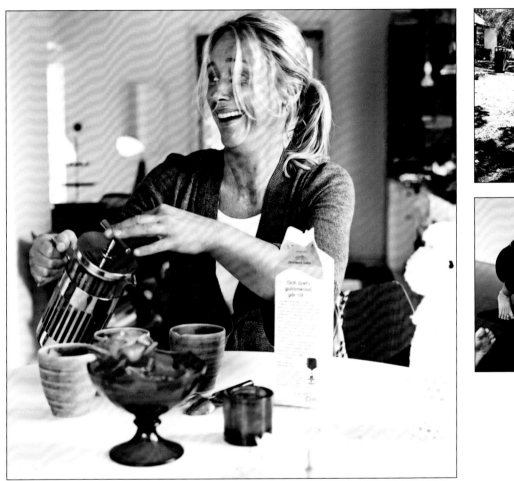
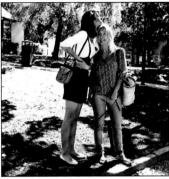
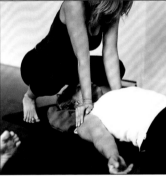

There are not really any specific rules to how to live a yogic life, if your goal is to become a yogini. But if you practice yoga often, you will soon want to eat healthier. At first you might make sure that everything that you put into your body is organic, then you might eliminate meat, then maybe fish. The craving for a glass of red wine on Friday night usually disappears, and many people stop drinking coffee. None of that is necessary to notice that the body feels good from practicing yoga, but many people find that it increases the sense of wellbeing.

Can anyone practice yoga?

I am convinced that anyone can practice yoga. Yoga can be adjusted to each individual's needs. You can choose a more physical type of yoga, or a more meditative style. I believe that breathing techniques and body stretches should be included into the school curriculum. You will notice quick results in both the young and the old. Already after a few classes, most people notice that they sleep better, feel happier, but first and foremost they start to care about their health and learn to listen to their own body.

As a teacher, I often encounter students that feel stiff and wonder if they will ever be able to sit in a lotus pose. They might be glancing at the flexible student with awe and jealously. I usually say that it is better to be stiff when you start out practicing, than to be overly flexible. The stiff person, if it is appropriate to use such a description, knows their limits. They possess a natural hindrance in their bodies and with the help of the breath and regular

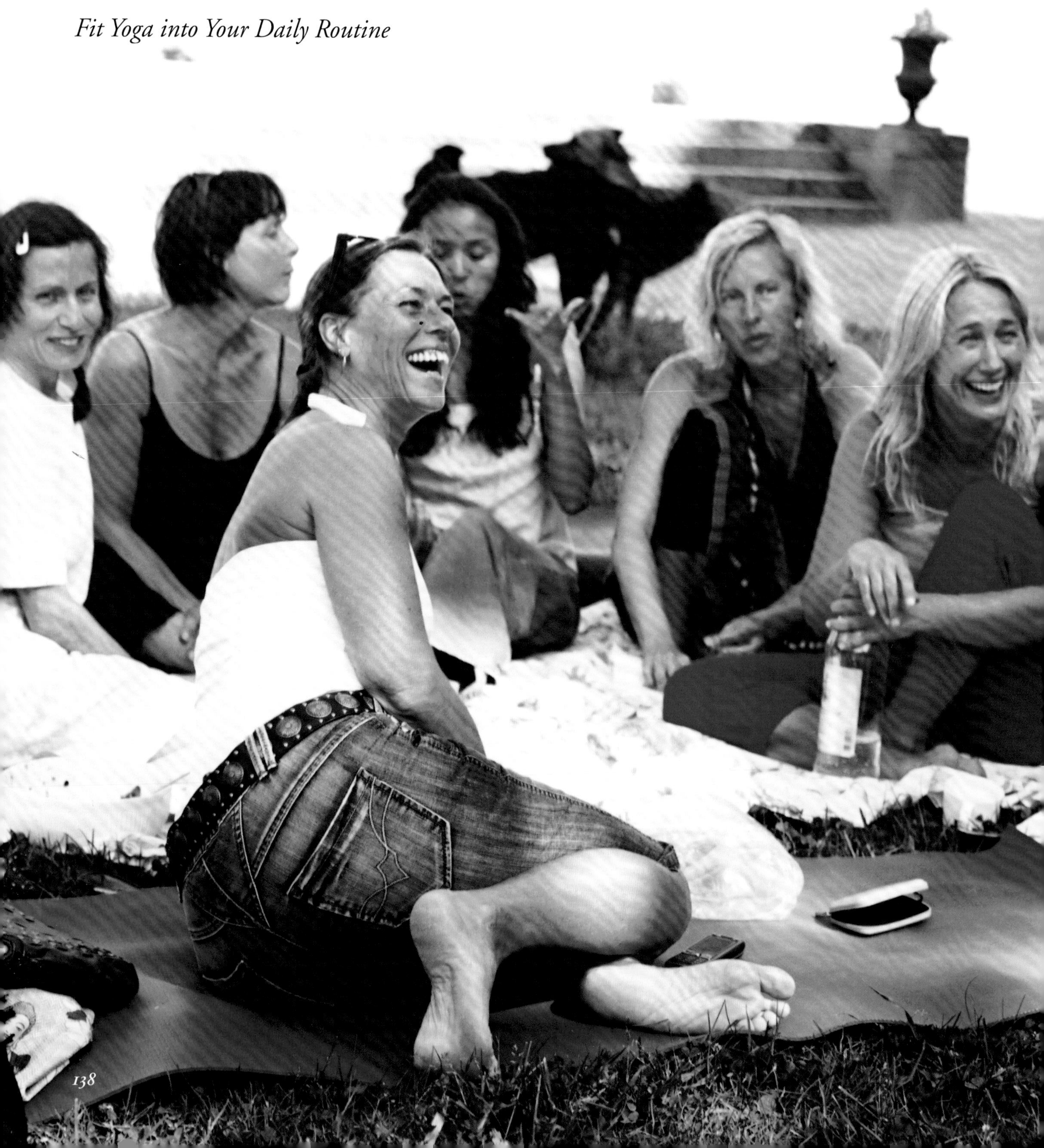

practice, that hindrance will soften and the person will become more flexible. The really flexible person, I am one of these people myself, has to learn about their own body. To be overly flexible can easily lead to injury. You get into a pose too easily, without engaging the muscles, and risk stretching the muscle off the bone. You need to find the strength and build up the muscles first. It can be difficult to take a step back and not fall into that flexible place.

One thing is for sure: Some people experience difficulties when they first start practicing yoga, but everyone encounters a tough point in their practice. It could be that you need to challenge one of your fears. I used to find headstands really scary. It took me a long time to learn to get into the pose. I still think it is a bit scary to stand on the hands. Other people might find it really fun and have done it since they were kids.

Yoga is a lifestyle. Yoga makes you more connected to yourself, to your body, and to your needs. To live a yogic life means to take care of oneself in the best possible way. If you greet each morning with five sun salutations, it proves that you put your wellbeing first and foremost. Get up a little bit earlier every morning, 15 minutes is enough. Light a few candles, maybe some incense. Roll out your mat and do a few sun salutations.

Don't forget that when we do something healing or good for somebody else, it is healing to us as well.

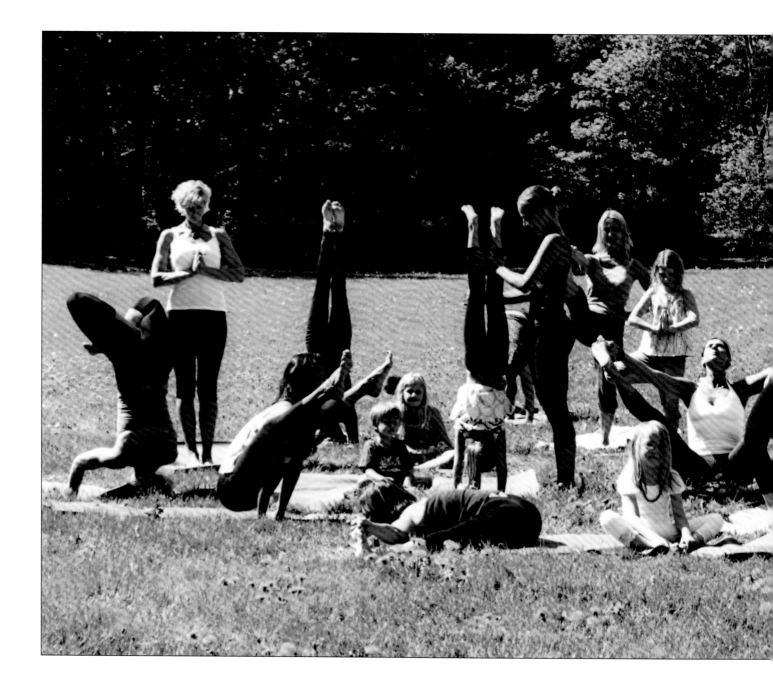

And when we do something good for ourselves, we also do it for other people. We all share the same energy field.

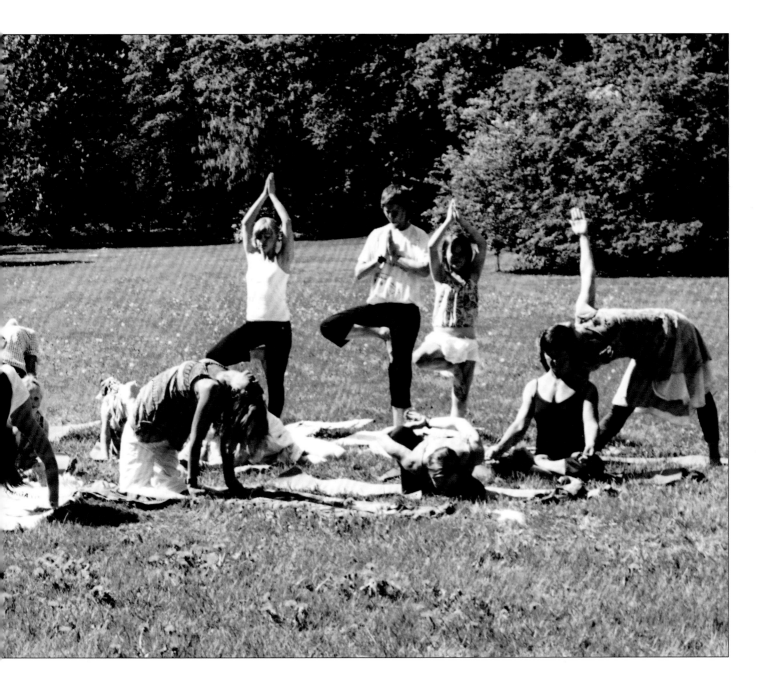

Index

Bibliography

Dancing the Body of Light, by Dona Hollema, Pegasus Enterprises

The Illustrated Encyclopedia of Healing Remedies, by C. Norman Shealy, Könemann Publishing

Ashtanga—Yoga Tradition of Sri K. Pattabhi Jois, by Petri Räisanen, Prisma Publishing

Yoga: The Path to Holistic Health, by B.K.S Iyengar

Yoga for Pregnancy, Birth and Beyond, by Françoise Barbira Freedman, B. Wahlström

Awakening the Spine, by Vanda Scaravelli, Harper Collins

The New Yoga for People Over 50, by Suza Francina, Health Communications, Inc

Yogini—The Power of Women in Yoga, by Janice Gates, Mandala

Moola bandha The Master Key, by Swami Buddhananda, Yoga Publications Trust

Hatha Yoga: The Hidden Language, by Swami Sivananda Radha, Jaico Book

Yoga and The Wisdom of Menopause, by Suza Francina, HCI Books

The New Yoga for People Over 50, by Suza Francina, HCI Books

Om Yoga, by Lisa Ljungh Strömberg, DN Publishing House

Yoga, Tantra and Meditation in Daily Life, by Swami Janakananda, Bindu

Ashtanga Yoga: The Complete Mind and Body Workout, by Juliet Pegrum, B. Wahlström

The Path of Yoga, by Osho, Energica Publishing House

The Seven Spiritual Laws of Yoga: A Practical Guide to Healing Body, Mind, and Spirit, by Deepak Chopra, Forum

Happy Yoga: 7 Reasons Why There's Nothing to Worry About, by Steve Ross, Energica Publishing House

Yoga Mind, Body & Spirit, by Donna Farhi, Owl Books

Centered Yoga, by Dona Holleman

Yoga Mala, by Sri K. Pattabhi Jois

Ashtanga Yoga, by Lino Miele